*To all of the healthcare workers
who have served on the front line during
the COVID-19 pandemic.
Bless you all for your dedication, devotion,
love, and compassion.*

MAX YOUR IMMUNITY

HOW TO MAXIMIZE YOUR IMMUNE SYSTEM WHEN YOU NEED IT MOST

PAMELA W. SMITH, MD, MPH, MS

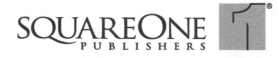

SQUAREONE
PUBLISHERS

The information and advice contained in this book are based upon the research and the personal and professional experiences of the author. They are not intended as a substitute for consulting with a healthcare professional. The publisher and author are not responsible for any adverse effects or consequences resulting from the use of any of the suggestions, preparations, or procedures discussed in this book. All matters pertaining to your physical health should be supervised by a healthcare provider.

Square One Publishers
115 Herricks Road
Garden City Park, NY 11040
(516) 535-2010 (877) 900-Book

Editor: Erica Shur
Cover and interior: Gary A. Rosenberg

Library of Congress Cataloging-in-Publication Data
Names: Smith, Pamela Wartian, author.
Title: Max your immunity : how to maximize your immune system when you need it most / Pamela Wartian Smith, M.D., MPH, MS.
Description: Garden City Park : Square One Publishers, [2021] | Includes index.
Identifiers: LCCN 2021015603 | ISBN 9780757005121 (paperback) | ISBN 9780757055126 (epub)
Subjects: LCSH: Nutrition. | Immunity—Nutritional aspects. | Natural immunity.
Classification: LCC RA784 .S5946 2021 | DDC 613.2—dc23
LC record available at https://lccn.loc.gov/2021015603

Printed in the United States of America

10   9   8   7   6   5   4

Contents

Acknowledgments

This book could not have been completed without the guidance of my editor, Erica Shur, of Square One Publishers. She listened to my many scientific explanations and skillfully helped me weave what I hope is a compelling and convincing message regarding the many ways you can enhance your immune system. I am deeply indebted to her for her patience.

I would like to thank my publisher, Rudy Shur, at Square One Publishers. Without him this book would not have been possible. I am the luckiest physician-author in the world to have the very best publisher in the world.

To my best friend and loving husband, Christopher, whose dedication to our family and his unwavering support of all of my activities have been instrumental in my ability to communicate to the world the importance of a Personalized Medicine approach to healthcare.

Introduction

Most people have become more interested in their health and even specifically in their immune system with the advent of the COVID-19 virus into the world. How can you build your immune system so that you do not develop this or other infectious diseases? If you do catch COVID-19, how do you maximize your immune system so that hopefully you do not have as severe a case of this potentially lethal illness?

The immune system is composed of specific cells and organs that ward off invaders. Normally it does a wonderful job of keeping you healthy and preventing infections and illnesses by guarding the body against everyday germs and microbes. Unlike many other parts of your body, where cells of various functions are located in areas that can be easily defined, the distribution of immune cells into various organs is more complicated. A great deal of research has recently focused on understanding the individual cell types within the immune system and identifying interacting cells and the messengers they use to communicate.

In this book, *Max Your Immunity*, you will learn proven therapies to increase your body's ability to fight off disease. In addition, you will discover how to restore and increase your immunity without developing an overactive immune system.

Part 1 of this book discusses the role your immune system plays. How does the immune system work? What are the innate and adaptive parts of the immune system? What are T cells, B cells, natural killer cells, and other cell lines you may not have heard of? What is an autoimmune disease? How is your immune system measured? Does you immune system change with age? All of these questions will be discussed at length in this section of the book.

It may surprise you that currently the number-one cause of disease in the United States and most industrialized countries is your immune system trying to protect you. It is all about balance. An overactive immune system leads to an autoimmune disease process. An underactive immune system leads to an increase in infection rate and risk of developing cancer. Furthermore, a variety of changes are observed in the immune system, which translate into less effective innate and adaptive immune responses and increased susceptibility to infections. The capability to cope with infectious agents and cancer cells resides not only in adaptive immune responses against specific antigens, mediated by T and B lymphocytes, but also in innate immune reactions. Moreover, an age-related decline in immune functions, referred to as immunosenescence, is partially responsible for the increased prevalence and severity of infectious diseases, and the low efficacy of vaccination in older individuals. In short, this section of the book provides a comprehensive reference map defining the organization and balance of the immune system.

Part 2 examines lifestyle changes and other considerations that can strengthen your immunity; from managing your stress, to optimizing gastrointestinal health, to minimizing sugar intake and alcohol intake, and a great deal more. Many of the ten keys discussed in this section can employed on your own without a healthcare provider's input. It is always best, however, to keep your doctor, or other healthcare professional, updated on changes in diet and other factors that you may implement to help heal and build your immune system.

Part 3 reviews herbal and nutritional therapies for building immunity. Research has shown repeatedly that nutritional deficiencies or inadequacies can cause your immune system not to function perfectly. Insufficient intake of micronutrients occurs for many reasons. In addition, new studies have shown that for certain nutrients higher doses may be needed to optimize immune functions, including improving immune defense and resistance to infection.

Likewise, many of these nutrients and herbal remedies help to maintain or improve immune function through different modalities of action; for example, inhibition of pro-inflammatory mediators, alteration of antigen-presenting cell function, anti-inflammatory action, modulation of cell-mediated immunity, as well as communication between the innate and adaptive immune systems. To be specific, micronutrient deficiencies suppress immune functions by affecting the innate T cell-mediated immune response and adaptive antibody response, which leads to an imbalance of the immune system. This increases your susceptibility to infections, along with an escalation in morbidity and mortality. Consequently, adequate intake of vitamins and minerals are required for the immune system to function efficiently.

Last, extensive sources of scientific studies, academic papers, and books have been used in writing *Max Your Immunity*. Therefore, you can review the medical literature on your own and also give a copy of this book to your healthcare provider in order to aid all in the worthwhile goal of optimizing your immune system.

PART 1

How Your Immune System Works

On a daily basis you breathe in thousands of foreign agents—viruses and bacteria—that travel around in the air from one person to another and can live on the surfaces of our environment. For the vast majority of time, your immune system handles all of these invaders without a problem and manages to protect you. How your immune system carries out its work is the subject of this section. Part 1 will explore the role the immune system plays in your body. It will provide you with a comprehensive explanation and understanding of the basics of the immune system. This section will also examine the various components of your immune system, how they work together and apart to protect you from infection, as well as what constitutes a healthy immune system.

You will learn what happens when your immune system becomes overreactive, which may lead to the development of an autoimmune disease. As you will see, there are many tests that can be performed by your healthcare provider to determine if your immune system is functioning optimally. Lastly, you will discover that your immune system can age as your body ages and learn ways to slow down this process.

This section is divided into four chapters:

1. What makes up your immune system?

2. What is an autoimmune disease?

3. How is your immune system measured?

4. Does your immune system change with age?

To say that your immune system can be explained in simple terms would be an overstatement. The fact is, this internal protection you have is made up of numerous cells that all work in different ways, but with the same purpose—to kill or disable these invaders. There is a lot of fascinating information in this section—however, while I have attempted to make it as understandable as possible, the processes involved are relatively complex. By first understanding the basics of your immune system, you will have a better idea of what you can do to strengthen your natural immunity while avoiding the most common invaders that seek to harm you. We will cover those areas in Part 2 and Part 3.

1

What Makes Up Your Immune System?

Different tissues work together in harmony to form complex systems in order to serve different vital functions in your body. The immune system is one of the most crucial systems. It encompasses tissues and cells that are associated with the defense of your body from different pathogens and infectious agents, such as viruses and bacterium. The immune system is generally classified into two different types: your innate immune system, also called the natural immune system, and your acquired immune system, also referred to as adaptive immunity. The purpose of both systems is to protect your body from disease or illness. In order to understand your immune system thoroughly, let us take a closer look at both of these systems in detail.

YOUR INNATE IMMUNE SYSTEM

Your innate immune system is designed to activate within minutes to hours after a foreign agent invades the body. Its purpose is to prevent the spread of harmful outside invaders. The innate immune system is composed of two lines of defense. The first line of defense consists of the skin, mainly the epidermis or outer skin, the gastric acid in the stomach, and the mucus membranes lining the tissues that are exposed to air, such as the nasal passages. The second line of defense consists of chemicals and cells that are released in the blood after being exposed to a pathogenic stimulus. The following is a summary of the characteristics of the innate immune system.

- These cells are active since birth, are operating all the time, and are ready to perform as soon as a foreign body enters your system.

- Once activated against a specific type of antigen, a toxin or foreign substance, the immunity remains throughout your life.

- It is inherited from your parents and passed down to your children.

- The response recognizes all types of pathogens, including, viruses, bacteria, and fungi.

- The same response is produced every time a pathogen invades the body.

- Its ability to fight off certain pathogens is limited.

YOUR ADAPTIVE IMMUNE SYSTEM

The adaptive system is mainly responsible for more complex reactions. This system activates after the innate response is fully implemented. Initially, the antigen entered in the body is identified by the specific immune cells, and then a cascade of reactions is started in the form of an antigen-antibody reaction to attack these outside invaders. This immune system also has the ability to remember these antigens, so that a specific response will be started should the same pathogen enter your body again in the future. The following is a summary of the characteristics of the adaptive immune system.

- These cells are normally in silent mode and become active only when the antigen is identified.

- The response is not immediate. It may begin to appear after a week or two after it has identified the outside invader. Consequently, it is called a delayed response type of immunity.

- The potency and effectiveness levels are very high since the combat cells the body generates are greatly specialized and also very powerful.

- The span of developed immunity lasts for a short time or may be lifelong.

- Unlike the cells of the innate immune system, these cells are not inherited.

- Each of these cells has a very specific purpose.

- Memory cells are present, which identifies specific cells on each exposure.

- The diversity of responses is very high.

Despite the differences, both immune systems have the same overall function—to protect you from harm. The innate response is produced initially for complete elimination of the pathogen, and then the delayed response is produced in the form of adaptive immunity—to continue to fight the battle and remember the identity of the invading enemy. Cells of both the systems coordinate equally to produce an effective and long-lasting response, protecting against harmful pathogens and infectious agents from entering the body. Furthermore, there are both similarities and differences between the cells produced by the innate and adaptive immune classifications.

Herd Immunity

Herd immunity is the resistance to the spread of an infectious disease within a population. It is based on pre-existing immunity of a high proportion of people due to previous infections and/or vaccinations. The percentage varies by disease. General estimates range from 80 percent to 94 percent of a group's population. *Acquired immunity* is established at the level of the individual, either through natural infection with a pathogen or through immunization with a vaccine. Thus, herd immunity is developed from the effects of individual (acquired) immunity scaled to the level of the population. The goal of herd immunity is to establish immunity so that those who cannot be vaccinated, such as very small children and immunocompromised individuals, are still protected against disease. The point at which the proportion of susceptible individuals falls below the threshold needed for transmission is called the *herd immunity threshold*.

The microbiome plays an essential role in helping your body develop immune cells for the emerging vaccination process whose goal is herd immunity. Frequency of interaction among microbiota, nutrients such as probiotics and prebiotics, as well as individual immunity preserve the degree of vaccine effectiveness. Microbiome symbiosis (the interaction between two different organisms which usually result in an advantage to both) regulates pathogen transmissibility and the success of vaccination among different age groups. Imbalance of good and bad bacteria, called dysbiosis, decreases immunity. Therefore, if your gut is not healthy (*see* chapter 7), you may be more vulnerable to the infection. Moreover, disparities of the protective response of many vaccines may be due to inconsistencies of healthy microbiota among individuals.

Consequently, herd immunity is the most critical and essential preventive intervention that delivers protection against once common diseases such as smallpox, polio, or measles. It has been made possible only because of natural vaccination through infection from the virus itself or expanded immunization programs.

CELLS OF THE INNATE AND ADAPTIVE IMMUNE SYSTEMS

The cells of both the innate and adaptive immune systems originate in the bone marrow which produces hematopoietic stem cells, that is, the cells that generate other blood cells. The hematopoietic stem cells then change into to two cell lines.

The myeloid cells. These cells can change into the red blood cells, platelets, neutrophils, eosinophils, basophils, and monocytes. The monocytes then make the dendritic cells and the macrophages. *This is your innate immune system.*

The lymphoid cells. Such cells give rise to natural killer cells, T lymphocytes, and B lymphocytes. *This is your adaptive immune system.* In addition, these cells also make other cells.

The T lymphocytes give rise to three types of cells.

1. Cytotoxic cells, also called killer T cells

2. Helper cells

3. Regulatory cells, also called suppressor T cells

The B lymphocytes give rise to plasma cells, which then produce antibodies.

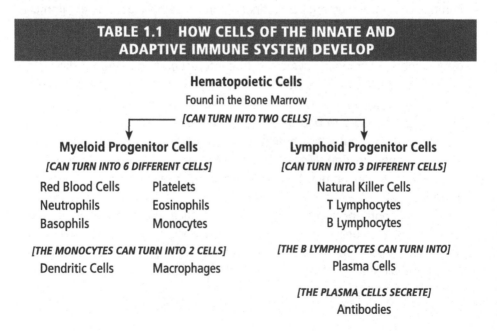

TABLE 1.1   HOW CELLS OF THE INNATE AND ADAPTIVE IMMUNE SYSTEM DEVELOP

Hematopoietic Cells
Found in the Bone Marrow
———— *[CAN TURN INTO TWO CELLS]* ————

Myeloid Progenitor Cells		**Lymphoid Progenitor Cells**
[CAN TURN INTO 6 DIFFERENT CELLS]		*[CAN TURN INTO 3 DIFFERENT CELLS]*
Red Blood Cells	Platelets	Natural Killer Cells
Neutrophils	Eosinophils	T Lymphocytes
Basophils	Monocytes	B Lymphocytes
[THE MONOCYTES CAN TURN INTO 2 CELLS]		*[THE B LYMPHOCYTES CAN TURN INTO]*
Dendritic Cells	Macrophages	Plasma Cells
		[THE PLASMA CELLS SECRETE]
		Antibodies

LYMPHOID CELLS

As discussed previously, the lymphoid cell line produces natural killer cells, B lymphocytes, and T lymphocytes. Let us examine each of these in depth.

Natural Killer Cells

Natural killer (NK) cells are lymphocytes of the innate immune system that control several types of tumors and microbial infections by limiting their spread and subsequent tissue damage. NK cell activation is controlled by a vibrant balance between the complementary and antagonistic pathways that are initiated upon interaction with potential target cells. NK cells express an array of activating cell surface receptors that can trigger cytolytic programs—a destruction of cells, as well as cytokine or chemokine secretion—protein signaling molecules that regulate immunity.

Furthermore, NK cells are also regulatory cells that engage in reciprocal interactions with the following:

- **Dendritic cells.** Cells that function as messengers within the innate and the adaptive immune systems.

- **Macrophages.** Cells that participate in identifying and destroying bacteria and other harmful organisms.

- **T cells.** Type of white blood cell (leukocyte) that holds a fundamental role in the immune system, also called T lymphocyte.

- **Endothelial cells.** Cells that line all blood vessels and control exchanges between the bloodstream and surrounding tissues.

Interestingly, natural killer cells can thus limit or exacerbate immune responses. Recent studies have shown that you can be born with a defect in three different genes that can cause a NK cell deficiency.

B Lymphocytes

B lymphocytes or B cells are a type of white blood cell of the lymphocyte subtype. They function in the humoral immunity component of the adaptive immune system by secreting antibodies. Additionally, B cells present antigens and secrete cytokines. B cells, unlike the other two classes of lymphocytes, T cells and natural killer cells, express B cell receptors (BCRs) on their cell membrane. BCRs allow the B cell to bind to a specific antigen, against which it will initiate an antibody response. There are several different types of B lymphocytes, including plasmablasts, plasma cells, lymphophasmacytoid cells, memory B cells, B-2 cell-F0 B cells, MZ B cells, B-1 cells, and regulatory B (B reg) cells.

T Lymphocytes

These white blood cells, T lymphocytes, that are essential to your immune system are divided into three groups of cells; helper T cells (Th1 and Th2), regulatory cells (suppressor T cells), and cytotoxic cells (killer T cells).

Helper T cells. The T helper cells (Th cells), also known as CD4$^+$ cells, are a type of T cell that play an important role in the immune system, particularly in the adaptive immune system. Helper T cells facilitate other cells in destroying harmful organisms. They also facilitate the activity of other immune cells by releasing T cell cytokines. Likewise, these cells help suppress or regulate immune responses. They are essential in helping to activate B cells to secrete antibodies and macrophages to destroy bacteria and viruses, in the activation and growth of cytotoxic T cells, and in maximizing bactericidal activity of phagocytes such as macrophages.

In addition, helper T cells are capable of influencing a variety of immune cells, and the T cell response generated (including the extracellular signals, such as cytokines) can be very important to help your body eradicate an infection. In order to be effective, helper T cells must determine which cytokines will allow the immune system to be most beneficial for the host.

Understanding exactly how helper T cells respond to immune challenges is currently of major interest in immunology, because such knowledge may be very useful in the treatment of disease and in increasing the effectiveness of vaccinations.

These cells come in two forms: Th1 and Th2. The following are the differences between the two types.

Type I/Th1

- The main partner cell types are macrophage and CD8+ T cells.

- The cytokines produced are interferon-y, TNF-B, interleukin-2, and interleukin-10.

- The immune stimulation promoted is from the cellular immune system. It maximizes the killing efficacy of the macrophages and the proliferation of cytotoxic CD8+ T cells. It also promotes the production of IgG which is an opsonizing antibody. Opsonization is the action in which specific antibodies in the blood attach to the exterior of a foreign antigen.

- Other functions include: The Type 1 cytokine IFN-y increases the production of interleukin-12 by dendritic cells and macrophages, and via positive feedback, IL-12 stimulates the production of IFN-γ in helper T cells, thereby promoting the Th1 profile. IFN-gamma also inhibits the production of cytokines such as interleukin-4, an important cytokine associated with the Type 2 response, and thus it also acts to preserve its own response.

Type 2/Th2

- The main partner cell types are B cell, eosinophil, and mast cells.

- The cytokines produced are interleukin-4, interleukin-5, interleukin-6, interleukin-9, interleukin-10, and interleukin-13.

- The immune stimulation promoted is from the humoral immune system. It stimulates B cells into proliferation, to induce B cell antibody class switching and to increase neutralizing antibody production (IgG, IgM, IgA, and IgE antibodies).

- Other functions include: The Type 2 response promotes its own profile using two different cytokines. Interleukin-4 acts on helper T cells to promote the production of Th2 cytokines, while interleukin-10 (IL-10) inhibits a variety of cytokines, including interleukin-2 and IFN-γ in helper T cells, and IL-12 in dendritic cells and macrophages.

There are also other types of helper cells that are produced in the body that are beyond the scope of this book.

Regulatory cells (Suppressor T cells), Suppressor T cells (Treg) (T8 or CD8+ cells) control the activity of other white blood cells so they do not destroy normal tissue. Specifically, Treg cells maintain order in the immune system by enforcing a dominant negative regulation on other immune cells. Broadly classified into natural or adaptive Tregs:

Natural Tregs are CD4+CD25+ T cells which develop and migrate from the thymus to perform their major role in immune homeostasis.

Adaptive Tregs are non-regulatory CD4+ T cells which acquire CD25 (IL-2R alpha) expression outside of the thymus, and are typically induced by inflammation and disease processes, such as autoimmune disorders and cancer.

The exact understanding of the entire immunosuppressive mechanism of T regulatory cells remains elusive.

Cytotoxic cells (Killer T cells). Killer T cells (a kind of CD8+ cell) recognize

The Magic of Cells

While you may have heard the term "stem cells" used, it is important to understand what that means in regard to the immune cells that we will be discussing. The body is composed of many different cells that all perform various tasks. From skin cells to blood cells to heart cells, each is there to carry on life-sustaining functions. Scientists have discovered that the stem calls in your body are unspecialized. That is, while they don't seem to have an obvious function, they are, in fact, fundamental to your existence.

In 1998, scientists discovered that by mixing stem cells with different combinations of proteins, they were able grow different types of specialized cells. In turn, with the right protein formulas they were able to turn these stem cells into heart, bone, kidney, nerve, and other specialized cells. It was later discovered that stem cells are found in every part of the body, and while stem cells may have a limited ability to diversify, we are still learning more about the potential of stem cells.

and destroy abnormal or infected cells. All viruses, and some bacteria, multiply in the cytoplasm of infected cells. Once inside cells, these pathogens are not accessible to antibodies and can be eliminated only by the destruction or modification of the infected cells on which they depend. Therefore, their role in host defense is fulfilled by cytotoxic CD8 T cells. Moreover, as well as controlling infection by viruses and cytoplasmic bacteria, CD8 T cells are important in controlling some protozoan infections. The elimination of infected cells without the destruction of healthy tissue requires the cytotoxic mechanisms of CD8 T cells to be both powerful and accurately kill infected targets with great precision along with sparing adjacent normal cells. This rigor is critical in minimizing tissue damage while allowing the eradication of infected cells.

CYTOKINES

Cytokines are a broad and loose category of small proteins important in cell signaling. Cytokine are peptides and cannot cross the lipid bilayer of cells so they cannot enter the cytoplasm. They are involved in three types of cell signaling:

- Autocrine signaling is a type of cell signaling where a cell discharges a hormone or chemical messenger (called the autocrine agent) that sticks to autocrine receptors on that same cell, which then leads to alterations in the cell.

- Paracrine signaling is a sort of cell signaling or cell-to-cell transmission in which a cell creates a signal to bring about changes in nearby cells, reshaping the behavior of those cells.

- Endocrine signaling takes place when endocrine cells discharge hormones that have an effect on distant target cells in the body.

Cytokines operate as agents of immune modulation—boosting the body's immune system—and are produced by many types of cells, including macrophages, B lymphocytes, T lymphocytes, mast cells, endothelial cells, fibroblasts, and various stromal cells. In addition, any cytokine can be produced by more than one kind of cell. Cytokines are important in health and disease, specifically in host immune responses to infection, inflammation, trauma, sepsis, and cancer. The following are different types of cytokines produced by the body.

- Chemokines control chemotaxis (movement of cells) and leukocyte recruitment. Many of these are proinflammatory.

- Colony-stimulating factors are involved with stimulation of hematopoietic progenitor cell (cells present in blood and bone marrow) proliferation and differentiation.

- Interferons regulate innate immunity. They have antiproliferative effects (prevent or slow down spread of cells). They also cause activation of antiviral properties by the body.

- Interleukins regulate growth and differentiation of leukocytes. Many of them are proinflammatory.

- Tumor necrosis factor is proinflammatory and it activates cytotoxic T lymphocytes.

Furthermore, adverse effects of cytokines have been linked to many disease processes, such as schizophrenia, depression, cancer, and Alzheimer's disease. Over secretion of cytokines can trigger a cytokine storm.

Cytokine Storm

Under normal circumstances, cytokines help coordinate the response of your immune system to take care of infectious substances, like viruses or bacteria. The problem is that sometimes the body's inflammatory response can get out of control, causing more harm than good. From time to time, the body produces too many inflammatory cytokines and not enough cytokines that modulate inflammation. Consequently, the inflammatory cytokines start "storming" out of control, without enough feedback from the anti-inflammatory cytokines.

Recent studies have shown that in people experiencing cytokine storm syndrome, certain cytokines are present in the blood at higher-than-normal amounts, which can cause multisystem organ failure and even death. In COVID-19, elevations in several inflammatory cytokines appear to be involved in the development of acute respiratory distress syndrome, the leading cause of death in people suffering with COVID-19.

Cytokine storms can be caused by a number of infectious and non-infectious etiologies including the following:

- Cytomegalovirus
- Epstein-Barr virus
- Group A streptococcus

- H5N1 influenza
- SARS-CoV-1
- SARS-CoV-2 which is COVID19

Individuals with certain autoimmune diseases may also have a higher risk of developing cytokine storm syndrome.

◼ Symptoms of Cytokine Storm Syndrome

Cytokine storm can cause many different symptoms. Sometimes these are only mild, flu-like symptoms. Other times, these can be severe and life-threatening. Symptoms may include:

- Confusion and hallucinations
- Cough
- Difficulty coordinating movements
- Fatigue
- Fevers and chills
- Headache
- Lethargy and poor responsiveness

- Muscle and joint aches
- Nausea and vomiting
- Rapid breathing
- Rash
- Seizures
- Shortness of breath
- Swelling of extremities
- Tremor

Very low blood pressure and increased blood clotting can also be hallmarks of severe cytokine storm syndrome. In addition, the heart may not pump as well as it normally would. As a result, cytokine storm can affect multiple organ systems, potentially leading to organ failure and death. New therapies are being developed all the time to decrease the inflammatory response. *See* the section on inflammation in Part 3 of this book.

HUMORAL AND CELL MEDIATED IMMUNITY

The adaptive system can further be divided into two categories: humoral immunity and cell-mediated immunity.

What are the *similarities* between humoral and cell mediated immunity?

● Humoral and cell mediated immunity are two types of adaptative immunity.

● Both immunity types activate upon the exposure to foreign antigens.

● They effectively defend your body against a variety of pathogens.

● Each of the immunities creates immunological memory against antigens.

● The mutual systems do not work correctly in immune-compromised individuals.

What is the *difference* between humoral and cell mediated immunity?

● The key difference between humoral and cell mediated immunity is the production of antibodies. Humoral immunity operates with antibodies produced by B lymphocytes, while cell mediated immunity does not involve antibodies.

● Humoral immunity mainly works against extracellular pathogens identified by the antibodies, while cell mediated immunity works against intracellular pathogens identified by the T cell receptors.

● Humoral immunity does not provide immunity against cancers, while the cell mediated immunity provides immunity against cancers.

In summary, there are two essential differences between humoral and cell mediated immunity. The key difference between these two immunities is that humoral immunity facilitates by the antibodies produced by B lymphocytes. In contrast, cell mediated immunity does not facilitate by the antibodies, it instead is mediated by Th cells and cytotoxic T lymphocytes. The other major difference between humoral and cell mediated immunity is that humoral immunity works against extracellular antigens, while cell mediated immunity works against intracellular antigens.

CONCLUSION

The predominant function of the immune system is to prevent or regulate infection. As you have learned in this chapter, the immune system is complex and extensive with a myriad of cell types that flow throughout your body performing a unique role. Each of the cell types have distinct ways of identifying problems, communicating with other cells, and carrying out their functions. When scientists better understand the workings of these cells, it allows them to confront specific health problems, extending from infections to cancer. I hope this chapter of Part 1 has given you a comprehensive, yet easily understandable, explanation of one of the most complex systems in your body: the immune system.

2

What Is an Autoimmune Disease?

Ahealthy immune system protects the body against infection and disease, however if an individual's immune system malfunctions, it can attack healthy cells, one or more tissues, or organs in your own body. Called autoimmune diseases, these attacks result in functional impairment, inflammation, and sometimes permanent tissue damage.

Autoimmune disease contributes substantially to states of depression and pain, excessive healthcare costs, and unfortunately, death. More than 50 million Americans are currently living with an autoimmune illness. Autoimmunity is the highest cause of morbidity in women in the United States and is one of the top ten causes of death in women under the age of 65. At least 85 percent of the cases of thyroiditis, systemic sclerosis, systemic lupus erythematosus, and Sjogren's syndrome patients are found in women.

Autoimmune diseases are frequently chronic illnesses, and it is estimated that more than 100 billion healthcare dollars are spent each year in the management of autoimmune patients, which places autoimmunity among the most-costly diseases to diagnose and treat. Although most maladies can occur at any age, some illnesses primarily occur in childhood and adolescence (such as type 1 diabetes), in the mid-adult years (for example, myasthenia gravis, multiple sclerosis), or among older adults (for example. rheumatoid arthritis, primary systemic vasculitis). Interestingly, the incidence of type 1 diabetes has increased, but the rates of rheumatoid arthritis have declined over the past 40 years.

WHAT CAUSES AUTOIMMUNE DISEASE?

To be more specific, autoimmune diseases are conditions in which your immune system mistakenly attacks your body. The immune system normally guards against bacteria, viruses, and toxins. When it senses these foreign invaders, it sends out an army of fighter cells to attack them. Normally, the immune system can tell the difference between foreign cells and your own cells. However, in an autoimmune disease, your system generates cellular and antibody responses to substances and tissues normally present in the body. As a result of this immune response, damage to different organs and tissues occurs. Autoimmune diseases can be either systemic or tissue-specific in nature; however, all forms of autoimmunity are thought to result from a disruption of balance within the immune system.

The precise cause of autoimmune diseases has not been identified. One existing hypothesis is that bacteria, viruses, or drugs may activate developments that confuse the immune system. This may happen more often in people who are genetically predisposed to autoimmune disorders.

Immunological Tolerance

The normal immune system is designed to recognize and react to a multitude of foreign pathogens while remaining unresponsive to host tissues (such as self-antigens). This ability to live with—or tolerate—self is called immunological tolerance. Generally, the immune system is tolerant of self-antigens, however when tolerance is absent disorders like autoimmune disease may arise.

Although lymphocytes specific for self-antigens are constantly being generated in the thymus (termed T lymphocytes or T cells), many of these cells are eliminated before they complete their maturation. However, this process is not perfect. Healthy individuals have circulating T cells that are capable of mounting pathogenic immune responses directed at self-antigens. However, most people do not develop an autoimmune disease. Instead, in healthy individuals, the pathogenicity of these self-reactive cells is counterbalanced by regulatory mechanisms that are constantly at work suppressing potentially damaging responses, thus maintaining tolerance to self.

AUTOIMMUNE DISEASE SYMPTOMS

There is no one set of symptoms that covers the range of autoimmune disease. The most common symptoms have a tendency to be nonspecific, in other words, they could be caused by a disorder that is not linked to the immune system. This ramification can make it more difficult for physicians to diagnose this type of condition. Despite the varying kinds of autoimmune diseases many of them may have similar signs and symptoms, which include:

- Abdominal pain or digestive issues
- Fatigue

- Joint pain and swelling
- Recurring fever
- Skin problems
- Swollen glands

Since there are different degrees of autoimmune disease, some people may experience milder symptoms, while they may be more severe for others. Certain diseases can also have their own distinctive symptoms. In addition, with autoimmune diseases like psoriasis or rheumatoid arthritis, one may experience a flare-up in which the symptoms may come and go.

RISK FACTORS

Autoimmune conditions affect people of all genders, races, and ages, however some people have an elevated risk of developing autoimmune disorders. The exact etiologies of autoimmune diseases have not been recognized although most researchers do believe that autoimmune diseases are due to an overactive immune system attacking the body after an infection, injury, or exposure to a toxin. If you have any of the following known risk factors, the probability of acquiring an autoimmune disorder is higher:

- Age: most autoimmune disorders affect younger people and middle-aged adults

- Certain medications

- Ethnicity: African Americans, Native Americans, or Hispanics are more likely to develop autoimmune disorders

- Excessive stress

- Exposure to environmental agents

- Gender: women are at higher risk for some autoimmune disorders

- Genetics: since some diseases tend to run in families

- Impaired intestinal barrier (The intestinal barrier allows for the intake of nutrients, electrolytes, and water, as well as antigens that play a role in immune regulation. A compromised intestinal barrier can lead to auto-immune disorders.)

- Infectious diseases have long been considered as one of the triggers for autoimmune and autoinflammatory diseases, mainly via molecular mimicry (structure of a molecule that imitates or stimulates the structure of a different molecule.)

- Obesity may be a risk factor for the development of some autoimmune diseases since being overweight is an inflammatory state.

- Smoking has been linked to several autoimmune processes.

There are a ways to decrease the accumulation of risk factors and help avert the beginnings of an autoimmune disorder. You can start by eating a nutritious diet and placing a limit on processed foods—try and eat organic foods as much as possible. Gluten intolerance is extremely common. It is characterized by an adverse reaction to gluten, which is a protein found in wheat and other grains. Celiac disease is an autoimmune disease where ingestion of gluten can literally damage the digestive system. All individuals with any autoimmune disease have an intolerance or sensitivity to gluten and should avoid all intake of gluten. In addition, integrate exercise and physical movement into your everyday life. Be aware of the current information about the medications you take and avoid cigarette smoking.

TYPES OF AUTOIMMUNE DISORDERS

There are over 100 autoimmune diseases that have been recognized and are being studied. They can act on any part of the body and come to be life-threatening. Some are well-known, such as type 1 diabetes, rheumatoid arthritis, and lupus, while various others are uncommon and a challenge to diagnose. The following are some of the more common autoimmune disorders:

- Alopecia areata
- Antiphospholipid syndrome
- Autoimmune hepatitis
- Celiac disease
- Chronic fatigue syndrome
- Chronic Lyme disease
- Crohn's disease
- Dermatomyositis
- Eczema (atopic dermatitis)
- Fibromyalgia
- Grave's disease
- Guillain-Barre syndrome

- Hashimoto's thyroiditis
- Multiple sclerosis
- Myasthenia gravis
- Parkinson's disease
- Pernicious anemia
- Polymyositis
- Primary biliary cirrhosis
- Psoriasis and psoriatic arthritis
- Rheumatoid arthritis
- Sarcoidosis
- Sjogren's syndrome
- Systemic lupus erythematosus (lupus)

- Systemic scleroderma
- Type I diabetes

- Ulcerative colitis
- Vitiligo

There are also implications of autoimmune pathology in such common health problems as arteriosclerosis, schizophrenia, and certain types of infertility.

CONVENTIONAL THERAPIES

In numerous autoimmune diseases, symptoms can approach remission with the appropriate drug therapy. These treatments zero in on avoiding symptom flare-ups. The most common treatment for autoimmune diseases, at this time, is immunosuppressive drugs. For many years steroids were the most frequently used medication, but they have been surpassed by immunosuppressive therapies due to the possible side effects of long-term steroid use.

Immunosuppressive Medications

Since autoimmune diseases are caused by immune cells attacking the host tissues they are supposed to protect. Recent advances suggest that maintaining a balance of effector and regulatory immune function is critical for avoiding autoimmunity. Therefore, traditional therapies for autoimmune disease have relied on immunosuppressive medications that systemically dampen immune responses.

These agents are highly effective for many patients and thus remain the current standard of care. However, long-term treatments with high doses are often needed to maintain disease control, leaving the person susceptible to life-threatening opportunistic infections and long-term risk of possibly developing other diseases, such as cancer. In addition, the benefits of many of these drugs are counterbalanced by toxicity and serious side effect profiles. Therefore, there has been a push for the development of more specific strategies that lower the risk of systemic immune suppression and improve tolerability.

Current Therapies Researched

New therapies, including regulatory T cell therapy, antigen-specific immunotherapy, manipulating the interleukin-2 pathway, and co-stimulation blockade all of which attempt to restore balance. Research has identified a host of co-signaling molecules that modulate the immune responses by T and B lymphocytes. Co-signaling molecules have been shown to have both positive and negative modulatory effects on T and B cell activation. In short, these approaches either focus on inhibiting the activation of pathogenic cells or are aimed at augmenting the pathways that naturally suppress these cells.

CONCLUSION

Beside traditional therapies, if you have an autoimmune process, the best place to begin is to avoid all gluten. This is for all autoimmune disease maladies, not just celiac disease. Furthermore, it is also important to optimize gastrointestinal health, and lastly to start low dose naltrexone (LDN). All of these therapies will be extensively discussed in other sections of this book. As you have seen, autoimmune diseases are a condition where your immune system attacks your own body. The goal of this book is to help you learn to maximize your immune system, but to also keep your body balanced so that you do not develop an autoimmune disease.

3

How Is Your Immune System Measured?

Laboratory studies are essential to determine the presence of a primary immunodeficiency disease. These tests are generally ordered by a physician when an individual experiences some type of inflammatory problem, such as a recurrent or chronic infection. Each cell type has a specialized function. As you have already learned in this section, the bone marrow produces hematopoietic stem cells, which then produce myeloid progenitor cells, which are part of the innate immune system. Hematopoietic stem cells also make lymphoid progenitor cells, which are part of the adaptive immune system.

In addition, blood tests can determine if you have normal levels of infection-fighting proteins called immunoglobulins in your blood. If you have too few immunoglobulins in your body, it gives you a greater chance of getting infections. Having too many may mean you have allergies or an overactive immune system.

MEASUREMENT OF THE INNATE IMMUNE SYSTEM

The laboratory measurement of the innate immune system is easily measured in the body by starting with a complete blood count (CBC). Each cell type has a specialized function. Eosinophils, basophils, and neutrophils are innate immune effectors—somewhat temporary activated cells—playing a key role in defense against pathogens. Red blood cells and platelet counts are also part of the results you receive when you have a complete blood count performed. In addition, monocytes are part of this test which produces macrophages and dendritic cells. These cells recognize pathogens and are essential in presenting antigens to initiate antigen-specific adaptive immune responses, thereby bridging the innate and adaptive immune systems.

MEASUREMENT OF THE ADAPTIVE IMMUNE SYSTEM

Lymphoid progenitor cells produce natural killer (NK) cells which are measurable by blood at any major laboratory. Lymphoid progenitor cells also produce B and T lymphocytes which moreover can be measured at any major lab.

Let us examine further each of these types of cells since they are not blood measurements that are routinely measured by your primary care provider. They are also discussed at length in the first part of this section, page 9. You can have any of these labs measured at a large laboratory, such as Quest or Lab Corp or any major hospital lab. Some of these studies are also measured by specialty labs that your doctor can arrange for you to have performed.

Natural Killer Cells

Natural killer (NK) cells are effector lymphocytes of the innate immune system that control several types of tumors and microbial infections by limiting their spread and subsequent tissue damage. Recent research highlights the fact that NK cells are also regulatory cells engaged in reciprocal interactions with dendritic cells, macrophages, T cells, and endothelial cells. NK cells can thus limit or exacerbate immune responses.

T Lymphocytes

T lymphocytes are the mediators of the adaptive cellular immune response as part of the cell-mediated immune response. Cell-mediated immunity is a response that does not involve antibodies. Theses mediators are also measured by a blood study, which can be done at any major laboratory. Some medications and other therapies can impact your T cell count and alter the accuracy of your test. The most common drugs that may affect your T cell count are: chemotherapy drugs, steroid use, and immunosuppressive drugs such as anti-rejection drugs. In addition, recent surgery or very stressful experiences can affect your T cell count as can radiation therapy. Let your healthcare provider know of any of these situations. T lymphocytes cells produce three types of cells all of which can be measured in the body by serum (blood), such as:

T helper cells. T helper cells (T4 or CD4 + cells) help other cells destroy harmful organisms.

Regulatory cells. Regulatory cells, now called suppressor T cells (T8 or CD8+ cells), control the activity of other white blood cells so they do not destroy normal tissue.

Cytotoxic cells. Cytotoxic cells, now called killer T cells (a kind of CD8+ cell), recognize and destroy abnormal or infected cells. When you go to the lab to have your blood drawn you will get all of the following results back if the entire T cell system is being measured.

- CD3+ absolute count represents the number of all T cells, which includes CD4 and CD8 cells.

- CD3 percentage represents the group of all immune cells that are T cells.

- CD4 cell count is the number of all CD4 cells.

- CD4 percentage represents the group of all T cells that are CD4 cells.

- CD8 cell count is the number of all CD8 cells, which includes both suppressor and killer T cells.

- CD8 percentage represents the group of all T cells that are CD8 cells.

- CD4/CD8 ratio (helper cell/suppressor cell ratio) is the number of the CD4 count divided by the CD8 count.

B Lymphocytes

B lymphocytes (plasma cells) are key effectors of the humoral immune response. Monocytes, dendritic cells, and B lymphocytes present antigens to T lymphocytes and play a central role in the development of the adaptive immune response. They also secrete cytokines. B cell lymphocytes do not attack and kill cells, viruses, or bacteria themselves. Instead, they manufacture proteins called antibodies that literally stick to the surface of invaders, disabling them, and highlighting them for clean up by other parts of the immune system. They can be measured as a blood study.

Dendritic Cells

Dendritic cells are a highly specialized white blood cell found in the skin, mucosa, and lymphoid tissues that initiate a primary immune response by activating lymphocytes and secreting cytokines. They are antigen-presenting cells. Their main function is to process antigenic material and present it on the cell surface to the T cells of the immune system. They furthermore act as messengers between the innate and adaptive immune systems.

Cytokines

Cytokines are small proteins which are important in cell signaling and immunomodulation. In addition, they are peptides and cannot cross the lipid bilayer of the cell and therefore cannot enter the cytoplasm. They are produced by many types of cells and can be produced by more than one type at a time, such as macrophages, B lymphocytes, T lymphocytes, mast cells, endothelial cells, fibroblasts, and stromal cells. Their concentrations vary during the course of a disease and in addition, cytokines can have both pro-inflammatory and anti-inflammatory effects. Cytokine assays are blood studies.

Immunoglobulins

The body produces several different immunoglobulins that are proteins with antibody activity that can be measured by your healthcare provider and are blood studies. They are part of the humoral immune response.

- Immunoglobulin A: IgA antibodies are found in the mucous membranes of the intestines, stomach, sinuses, and lungs. They are also found in the saliva, tears, and the blood.

- Immunoglobulin G: IgG is the most common type of antibody your body produces. These help to protect you against an infection by remembering which germs you have been exposed to in the past. If they return, your immune system will attack them.

- Immunoglobulin M: IgM is made by your body when you are first infected from a new bacteria or virus. Levels then begin to decline as your IgG levels become elevated and increase to protect you long-term.

- Immunoglobulin E: IgE levels increase when you are exposed to pollen or other items that you are allergic to.

- Immunoglobulin D: IgD levels are found in trace amounts and serve as a B lymphocyte surface receptor.

CONCLUSION

As you have seen in this chapter, the science is now here to measure many facets of your complex immune system. New tests and testing methods are now available to help examine your immune system in a more comprehensive manner than would have been possible only a few years ago.

4

Does Your Immune System Change With Age?

Do you find you get ill more often than you did when you were younger? When you are ailing, does it take a longer time to recover? As you age, your immune system ages as well, and it becomes evident that there is an increasing deterioration in your capacity to respond to vaccines efficiently. Because of this, you are more likely to get sick and to recuperate from injuries, infection, and disorders at a slower pace. Since there is no predetermined age when immunity decreases, it is crucial to go to the doctor routinely, and get medical support if you get sick frequently or if you're having difficulty healing after injury or illness. Research has shown that a decline in immune function is the most recognized effect of aging.

IMMUNOSENESCENCE

Given the consequential clinical indications of the changed immune status in aged people, it is of utmost importance to recognize, the essence of, and workings responsible for immunosenescence. Immunosenescence refers to the gradual deterioration of the immune system brought on by the aging process which translates into less effective innate and adaptive immune responses and increased susceptibility to infections, cancer, chronic inflammatory disorders, and autoimmune diseases. The capability to cope with infectious agents and cancer cells resides in the adaptive immune responses against specific antigens and mediated by T and B lymphocytes.

T cell functional dysregulation is a biomarker for immunosenescence. The functional capacity of T cells is the most influenced by the effects of aging. In fact, age-related alterations are evident in all stages of T cell development, making them a significant factor in the development of immunosenescence.

This situation leaves the body practically devoid of virgin T cells, which makes you more prone to a variety of infectious and non-infectious diseases as the years go by. Innate immune dysregulation also occurs over time. These innate defense mechanisms include chemotaxis, phagocytosis, natural cytotoxicity, cell interactions, and cytokines production.

Influence of Aging

With age, many individuals do not show signs and symptoms of their infection or disease process, which leads to a possible issue with expedient diagnosis and treatment. Likewise, as you age, changes in the immune system can occur, for example:

- Accumulation and the expansion of memory and effector T cells

- Alteration in granulocytes

- Alterations in the expression and function of adhesion molecules, which results in an augmented capacity to adhere

- Antigen-presenting function of dendritic cells is known to diminish which causes a deficiency in cell-mediated immunity and thus the inability for effector T lymphocytes to promote an adaptive immune response.

- Changes in cytokine profile, for example, an increase in pro-inflammatory cytokines

- Changes in intracellular signal transduction capabilities

- Changes in natural killer cell function, such as:
  - Change in anti-microbial immune response
  - Change in eliminating transformed cells
  - Decrease in recognition and elimination of senescent cells
  - Decrease in the ability to regulate the immune system
  - Decrease in the secretion of immunoregulatory cytokines and chemokines
  - Decreased cytotoxicity with increased incidence of bacterial and fungal infections
  - Increased reactivation rates of latent Mycobacterium tuberculosis
  - Slower resolution of inflammatory responses

- Decline in both the production of new naive lymphocytes and the functional competence of memory cell populations

- Decline in humoral immunity caused by a reduction in the population of antibody producing B cells along with a smaller immunoglobulin diversity and affinity

- Decreased ability to produce effector lymphokines

- Decrease in the total number of phagocytes with a reduction of their bactericidal activity

- Decreased production of cytokines and lower cytotoxicity

- Hampered immune defenses against viral pathogens, especially by cytotoxic CD8+ T cells

- Hematopoietic stem cells decrease their ability to renew themselves. This is due to the accumulation of oxidative damage to DNA by the aging process and cellular metabolic activity as well as the shortening of the telomeres on chromosomes.

- Impaired development of CD4+ T follicular helper cells. These cells:
  - Generate antibody-producing plasma cells
  - Produce memory B cells
  - Specialize in facilitating peripheral B cell maturation
  - Impaired proliferation in response to antigenic stimulation
  - Macrophages become dysregulated as a consequence of environmental changes
  - Neutrophils often exhibit a diminished phagocytic capacity and depressed respiratory burst
  - Reduction in the CD4+/CD8+ ratio
  - Th1 to Th2 cytokine production shifts and an increase in production of proinflammatory cytokines occurs
  - Shrinkage of antigen-recognition repertoire of T cell receptor diversity

Influence of Stress

In addition, immunosenescence may be significantly influenced by psychological stress and related stress hormones. In fact, there are similarities between immunosenescence and stress-related immunological changes. Medical trials have suggested possible links between endocrine senescence (endocrine changes with aging) and immunosenescence. Whereby age-related increases in inflammatory cytokines affect the release of hormones and, vice versa, hormonal changes associated with aging influence cytokine networks. Moreover, it has long been known that proinflammatory cytokines can readily activate the hypothalamic-pituitary-adrenal (HPA) hormonal axis during infection and after cytokine administration.

Likewise, chronic stress during aging leads to accelerated immunosenescence for both the patient and their caretaker. Markers of inflammation, such as IL-6 and c-reactive protein (CRP), may increase as well as NF-kB which is an important proinflammatory transcription factor. Consequently, chronic stress has been shown to lead to premature aging of the T cells of the immune system.

Influence of Environmental and Lifestyle Factors

As you have seen, immunosenescence is characterized by its high prevalence, individual variability, and complexity. In other words, the immune system is not uniformly affected by the aging process. New studies are suggesting that part of this personalized immune response that occurs with aging is that immunosenescence is not only the result of aging, but rather is also due to secondary changes caused by environmental and lifestyle factors. Nutrition, exercise, and even medications taken during your life can influence immune function as you age.

Over time, the epithelial barriers of the skin, lungs, and digestive tract break down, and make you more susceptible to pathogens. On a cellular level, immune cells, such as T cells and B cells, behave differently in the aging body. Likewise, the ability of these cells to respond to the threat of foreign bodies is decreased, increasing the risk of developing infections, such as influenza, pneumonia, and even COVID-19. In addition, immunosenescence not only affects the immune system's ability to protect against disease but also has a suppressant effect on vaccines, making them less effective as the years accrue.

CONCLUSION

While people are living longer, the increase in longevity does not always coincide with the increase in healthspan—healthy years living a quality of life. As a way of counteracting the effects of immunosenescence, healthcare providers may recommend a comprehensive healthy eating program, exercise, vitamins and herbal supplements, hormone replacement therapy, and perhaps even the administration of multiple doses of vaccines to boost their effectiveness. Tips on living a healthy lifestyle, and herbal and nutritional therapies, to help immune building are found in Part 2 and Part 3 of this book.

PART 2

Lifestyle Changes to Strengthen Your Immunity

Part 2 of this book examines lifestyle changes that can strengthen your immunity. Most of these ten key strategies you can employ on your own without a healthcare provider's input. It is always best, however, to keep your doctor or other health professional updated on changes in diet, nutrients, and other things that you are doing to help heal and build your immune system.

As we discussed in Part 1, your innate immune response is your body's existing defenses against foreign invaders, referred to as pathogens. Your adaptive immunity response is the secondary defensive response created independently to bolster and/or fight the invading pathogens.

This section covers these ten key strategies:

- Alcohol: Moderation is the Key to Good Health
- Exercise: Whether You Like It or Not

- Gut: A Healthy Gut Equals a Healthy Immune System
- Inflammation: Its Effect On the Immune System
- Sleep: Get a Good Night's Sleep
- Smoking: How It Affects the Immune System
- Stress: Manage Your Stress
- Sugar: Minimize Your Intake
- Thyroid: Optimize Its Function
- Water: Stay Hydrated

These sections will help you understand the ways to maximize your immune system and help balance the functions in your body so that it performs optimally.

5

Alcohol
Moderation Is the Key to Health

Some people can enjoy a glass of wine with food and drink moderate amounts of *alcohol* in social settings without any problems. However, as you will see, there is conflicting data regarding mild consumption of alcohol and your health. Even though millions of Americans, on average, consume 10 to 11 drinks weekly, many people don't appreciate the degree to which it may harm your body. Excessive drinking, which includes binge drinking and heavy drinking, particularly, can take a heavy toll on your physical as well as mental health in the long run. Alcohol abuse can negatively influence multiple pathways of the immune response, leading to an increased risk of developing infections. The course and resolution of both bacterial and viral infections are severely impaired in alcohol-abusing individuals, which also results in greater morbidity and mortality.

Consequently, specific changes in innate immune response and abnormalities in adaptive immunity caused by excessive alcohol intake are discussed in this chapter. In addition, altered inflammatory cell and adaptive immune responses after alcohol consumption can result in increased incidence of infection and poor outcome as well as other organ-specific immune-mediated effects. These processes involve structural host defense mechanisms in the gastrointestinal and respiratory tract, as well as the principal components of the innate and adaptive immune systems, which are compromised both through alcohol's direct and indirect effects.

EFFECTS OF ACUTE AND CHRONIC ALCOHOL ABUSE

If you are a little excessive in your alcohol consumption occasionally, it probably will not result in any long-term harm if you are otherwise healthy. But it's a different scenario if you consistently drink too much. Alcohol makes it more difficult for the immune system to be prepared to defend the body against harmful germs and serious infections. As you will see, chronic alcohol abuse compromises the immune system and various parts of the body in a number of ways. It can also alter the actions of cell populations in the innate and adaptive immune responses.

Effects on the Immune System

Immediate and chronic alcohol use has major immune effects on the body. Cells of the innate immune system, including NK cells, macrophages, monocytes, and dendritic cells, are weakened by alcohol in their capacity to respond to pathogens that present to your body. In addition, inflammatory cell responses including production of pro-inflammatory cytokines, such as (IL-1, TNF-alpha) and NF-kB activation, are inhibited by acute alcohol exposure, while chronic use of alcohol increases these pro-inflammatory responses. Likewise, the antigen presenting function of both monocytes and dendritic cells is impaired by both acute and chronic alcohol use and this contributes to impaired production of adaptive immune responses. In addition, both acute (immediate) and chronic use of alcohol inhibits T cell functions and IL-12 production and results in alterations in Th1 and Th2 cytokine production. Abuse of alcohol also has a major effect on B cell function by decreasing the number and function of the B cells, which results in a reduced capacity to generate protective antibodies in the body, including the mucous membranes. These abnormalities caused by alcohol use then together contribute to impaired elimination and reduced adaptive immune responses. These affects can have a negative effect on many organs of the body leading to a compromised immune system and an increased susceptibility to other diseases.

Effects on the Gut and Liver

Alcohol abuse may give rise to bacteria overgrowth in your gut which can in time travel through the intestinal wall and into the liver, leading to liver damage. It is the liver's task to draw out toxins, like alcohol, however your liver may not be able to function optimally if you suffer from chronic abuse. Alcohol can literally destroy liver cells. It leads to excessive intestinal permeability which decreases the immune system. This results in a chronic inflammatory environment conducive to liver injury. Long-term abundant use of alcohol may lead to scarring called cirrhosis and to fatty liver disease.

Effects on the Lungs

In the lungs, alcohol damages the immune cells that have the important job of cleaning out pathogens from our airways. Alcohol abuse also has a negative effect upon the lung respiratory system by decreasing the levels of the anti-oxidant glutathione in the lung, leading to oxidative injury. In addition, the ciliated epithelium—fine hairs—of the airways is impaired by alcohol, which increases the risk of airborne bacteria entering the lungs contributing to the increased risk of infection associated with excessive alcohol abuse.

Furthermore, alcohol abuse suppresses the production and secretion of some acute-phase proteins. This effect may contribute to lung injury in response to inflammation. Similarly, excessive drinking is linked to pneumonia and other pulmonary diseases.

ALCOHOL AND CANCER

As specified by the American Cancer Society, there may be a direct link between heavy alcohol use and many types of cancer. Alcohol alters the composition of your gut microbiome, and by damaging those cells you decrease your body's defense mechanism. This can lead to bacterial and viral infections, and a negative impact of alcohol on the immune system can precipitate an increased risk of cancer. It may put you at risk for some cancers such as:

- Breast
- Colon and rectum
- Esophagus
- Liver
- Mouth
- Larynx (voice box)
- Pharynx (throat)
- Stomach

HOW MUCH IS TOO MUCH?

According to the guidelines for Americans, moderate or mild drinking is defined as one drink per day for women and up to two drinks per day for men. Excessive drinking (described as more than one drink per day for women and more than one or two drinks per day for men) has been proven to be linked to an increased risk for many health issues. Problematic drinking or heavy alcohol use is defined as binge drinking, consuming excessive alcohol five or more days a month, which can lead to a physical dependency negatively impacting your health and your life.

Research has clearly shown that excessive drinking weakens your immune system making you more susceptible to various forms of cancer and other health issues. The question of moderate consumption is much more complicated. Medical trials have shown mild consumption of alcohol, in some cases, is associated with reduced inflammation and improved immunity. This may be due to alcohol's ability to lower stress levels. However, for some people it can increase the odds of developing various forms of cancer, such as breast cancer (*see* the inset on page 36).

Alcohol Use and Breast Cancer Risk

The results of many studies suggest that alcohol consumption may be associated with an increase in breast cancer risk in women. Unlike other forms of cancer, in this case drinking even small amounts of alcohol is linked with an increased risk of breast cancer. Overall, the amount of alcohol someone drinks over time, not the type of alcohol beverage seems to be the most important factor in raising cancer risk. It does not matter therefore, if the alcohol is in the form of beer, wine, or distilled spirits or other drinks according to medical studies.

Alcohol can raise estrogen levels in the body, which may explain some of the increased risk. Daily alcohol consumption increases serum estrogen levels, particularly estrone (E1) but also estradiol (E2) and other forms of estrogen. In fact, alcohol consumption increases the risk of breast cancer in estrogen receptor (ER)-positive tumors in postmenopausal women in several studies. This hypothesis is further supported by data showing that the alcohol-breast cancer association is limited to women with estrogen-receptor positive tumors. One study revealed that among healthy postmenopausal women who were not on hormone replacement therapy and who consumed 15 to 30 grams of alcohol per day, concentrations of estrogen (E1) were increased. Similarly, alcohol intake after breast cancer diagnosis is associated with both an increased risk of recurrence and also death.

Another trial revealed that alcohol not only increases estrogen, but also interferes with estrogen pathways by affecting estrogen receptors. It also showed how alcohol can negatively affect folate levels, and that folate changes affects DNA methylation and DNA synthesis, which is important

CONCLUSION

As the science has shown too much alcohol can have many devastating effects on your health. One of the least appreciated medical complication of alcohol abuse is altered immune regulation leading to immunodeficiency and autoimmunity (the immune system acts against its own tissues). The consequences of the immunodeficiency include increased susceptibility to bacterial pneumonia, tuberculosis, and other infectious diseases.

Current research on the altered cytokine balance produced by alcohol is leading to new insights on the regulation of the immune system in individuals that abuse alcohol. Furthermore, recent development of exciting new in the development of cancer. Furthermore, other studies have shown that genetic variants of one-carbon metabolism genes might increase alcohol-related breast cancer risk.

Moreover, mounting evidence suggests that antioxidant intake, for example folate, may reduce alcohol-associated breast cancer risks because it neutralizes reactive oxygen species, a second-stage product of alcohol metabolism. Therefore, diets lacking sufficient antioxidant intake may further elevate the risk of breast cancer among women consuming alcohol. Moreover, studies have shown that chronic alcoholism leads to folate deficiency which also contributes to the development of alcoholic liver disease. Furthermore, the intestinal absorption of folic acid was decreased in binge drinking alcoholics and, prospectively, in volunteers fed alcohol with low folate diets. To be specific, chronic alcohol exposure impairs folate absorption by inhibiting expression of the reduced folate carrier and decreasing the liver uptake and kidney conservation of circulating folate. At the same time, folate deficiency accelerates alcohol-induced changes in hepatic (liver) methionine metabolism while promoting enhanced oxidative liver injury and the development of liver disease.

As you have seen, alcohol intake alters immune function in the body and with the additional research showing that alcohol intake increases the risk of breast cancer in women through other mechanisms, more research needs to be done concerning the risk factors for breast cancer in women and its relationship to alcohol use. In the meantime, building your immune system by using all of the suggestions in this book along with decreasing alcohol intake is suggested to help lower breast cancer risk in women.

techniques designed to improve or restore immune function by manipulation of cytokine balance are being studied. Consequently, as you have seen, analyses of alcohol's diverse effects on various components of the immune system provide insight into the considerations that lead to a greater risk of infection in the alcohol-abusing population.

Chronic heavy drinking is associated with a decreased frequency of lymphocytes and increased risk of both bacterial and viral infections and literally compromises the immune response in many different ways. Moderation is the key to health! However, with this said, it is important you consider your family's health history.

6

Exercise
Whether You Like It or Not

Disciplined, consistent exercise is linked to significant benefits in your overall immune system health—the body's defense against infections. In the short-term, exercise aids the immune system in detecting and tackling viruses and bacteria; in fact, lack of activity is an independent risk factor for more than twenty-five chronic diseases. Over the long-term, regular exercise decelerates the changes that occur to the immune system.

Regarding the direct effect on the immune system, moderate exercise seems to exert a protective effect, whereas repeated bouts of strenuous exercise can result in compromised immune function along with an elevation in the stress hormone cortisol and the neurotransmitter epinephrine. Consequently, exercise in moderation is one of the keys to a healthy immune system. True exercise is defined as doubling your pulse for 20 minutes.

This chapter will discuss the affects that exercise has on the immune system in relationship to lack of exercise, the right amount of exercise, vigorous exercise, and very vigorous exercise programs. Regular physical activity exerts a multitude of beneficial health effects but, perhaps more importantly, is its ability to both enhance immune defense and mitigate the deleterious effects of stress on immunity.

The fact of the matter is that we live in an increasingly sedentary society, since modern technology and longer hours at desk jobs (whether at home or the workplace) have made it less necessary (and less convenient) to be physically active. The annual National Health Interview Survey found that only 35 percent of adults over the age of eighteen engage in some kind of physical activity on a regular basis. A staggering one-third of adults do not engage in any activity at all. These statistics reflect the alarming—and rising—rates of obesity, diabetes, and heart disease in the United States and all developing nations, not to mention high blood pressure, elevated cholesterol levels, and change in immune function.

WHAT IS EXERCISE?

There is an important distinction between physical activity and exercise. Physical activity is a general term that can be applied to any movement that engages the muscles, ranging from daily chores such as gardening, making beds, or vacuuming, to rigorous sports like tennis, running, or swimming, which raise the heart rate and build endurance. The term exercise, however, refers to planned, purposeful movement specifically intended to boost physical fitness. Running, walking, biking, swimming, sports, hot yoga, and dancing are all activities that require effort, expend energy, and work core muscle groups.

Aerobic Vs Anaerobic Exercise

Exercise is divided into two main categories; aerobic and anaerobic. Aerobic exercise (which is also called cardiovascular exercise) includes any activity that is rhythmic, continuous, and prolonged, and therefore increases your heart rate and requires additional intake of oxygen. Running, cycling, swimming, skating, aerobic dancing, climbing stairs, and jumping rope are all forms of aerobic exercise.

Anaerobic exercise, on the other hand, requires very little increase in oxygen, as it is typically shorter in duration and of higher intensity. Weightlifting, sprinting, jumping, rowing, doing push-ups, doing sit-ups, and serving volleyballs or tennis balls are all examples of anaerobic exercise. These activities are generally strenuous, involve quick bursts of energy, and result in muscle fatigue rather than oxygen deficit.

Although anaerobic exercise builds strength and lean muscle mass, aerobic exercise is what health organizations like the American College of Sports Medicine (ACSM) are generally referring to when they give their recommendations for physical activity. According to the ACSM, American Health Association, and Surgeon General, adults need about 30 minutes of moderately intense cardiovascular activity (aerobic exercise) four or five days a week, or 20 minutes of vigorous cardiovascular activity three times a week.

BENEFITS OF EXERCISE

Regular exercise is one of the most vital tasks for your well-being and good health. All of us can experience the health benefits of exercise, regardless of age, sex, physical abilities, ethnicity, shape, or size. The following are the benefits that exercise has on both your body and mind:

- Anti-inflammatory influence
- Blood pressure control
- Decreases susceptibility to depression or anxiety
- Enhances mood
- Enhances the immune system
- Exercise in the morning improves sleep
- Helps maintain memory
- Improves mobility and balance
- Increases self-esteem
- Lowers elevated blood sugar
- Modulator of intestinal microbiome composition
- Promotes weight loss
- Sleep

In addition, physical activity/exercise has been reviewed in the medical literature as being a primary way of preventing over 30 chronic conditions and premature death, such as:

- Anxiety
- Breast cancer
- Chronic pain
- Cognitive decline/Alzheimer's disease
- Colon cancer
- Congestive heart failure
- Constipation
- Coronary heart disease
- Deep vein thrombosis
- Depression
- Diverticulitis
- Endometrial cancer
- Erectile dysfunction (ED)
- Gallbladder disease
- Gestational diabetes
- Hypertension (high blood pressure)
- Insulin resistance
- Irritable bowel disease
- Metabolic syndrome
- Nonalcoholic fatty liver disease
- Obesity
- Osteoarthritis
- Osteopenia/Osteoporosis
- Peripheral artery disease
- Polycystic ovarian disease (PCOS)
- Pre-diabetes
- Pre-eclampsia
- Rheumatoid arthritis
- Sarcopenia
- Stroke
- Type 2 diabetes

Exercise has a variable effect on the immune system. If you do not exercise or only exercise occasionally, your immune system may be compromised. If you exercise the right amount it builds your immune system, and if you exercise vigorously daily it can compromise your immune system. Let's examine all three scenarios.

LACK OF EXERCISE

Multiple studies have demonstrated the profound impact that exercise can have on the immune system. However, the physical and psychological indicators of insufficient exercise go beyond just a decreased immune system. Some of the symptoms associated with lack of physical activity include:

- Cognitive decline
- Knee pain
- Lack of mobility
- Loss of balance, especially in the elderly
- Loss of flexibility
- Low self-esteem

- Muscle strain
- Poor muscle tone
- Proneness to injury
- Sleep apnea and other sleep disorders
- Susceptibility to depression or anxiety
- Weakened immune system

If you have not been exercising, then see your primary care doctor for a physical exam if you are over the age of 40 before you begin an exercise program.

EXERCISE THE RIGHT AMOUNT

Exercising the right amount is 3 to 4 times a week, doubling your pulse for 20 minutes which has many positive effects upon the body. One of the little-known benefits of exercise is that it boosts your immune system by reducing chronic low-grade infection, improving various immune markers, and also improving your response to vaccinations.

Clinical trials have also revealed that individuals that are physically active are less likely to report symptoms of upper respiratory illness. In addition, there is evidence that exercise can protect a person from many types of viral infection, including influenza, rhinovirus (another cause of the common cold), and the reactivation of latent herpesviruses, such as Epstein-Barr (EBV), varicella-zoster (VZV), and herpes-simplex-virus-1 (HSV-1).

A good exercise program also helps you to have better control over latent viral infections, even if you have times when you are confined to home. Latent viral reactivation is a hallmark of compromised immunity, which may be associated with isolation and inactivity as a result of confinement. In fact, long periods of isolation and confinement elevate cortisol levels (*see* chapter on cortisol) that can inhibit many critical functions of your immune system, such as the ability of lymphocytes to multiply in response to infection and the effector functions of NK cells and CD8+ T cells, all of which are needed for the recognition and elimination of viruses.

HOW EXERCISE IMPROVES YOUR IMMUNE SYSTEM

Exercise in the short-term helps the immune system to locate and control foreign invaders, and in the long-term it decelerates the changes that occur to the immune system with aging. The immune system benefits from exercise due to frequent mobilization and redistribution of effector lymphocytes, white blood cells—natural killer cells, T cells, and B cells.

Billions of lymphocytes are mobilized in response to a single bout of exercise, such as the mobilization of catecholamine-mediated subtypes are capable of tissue migration primed to recognize and kill virus-infected cells. Virus-specific memory T cells mobilized with exercise exhibit enhanced proliferation responses to viral antigens, such as those derived from CMV, EBV and HSV-1, and dormant viruses such as adenovirus—common viruses that cause a range of illness (cold-like symptoms, fever, sore throat, pneumonia). This process is also vital to minimize the impact of the virus and to expedite viral resolution should your immune barriers be breached and you become infected.

Exercise also releases various cytokines (interferon, interleukin) from the skeletal muscle (for example, myokines—small proteins) that can help maintain immune competency. Muscle-derived IL-6 has been shown to direct immune cell trafficking towards areas of infection. IL-7 can stimulate T cell production from the thymus and IL-15 helps maintain T cell and NK-cell homeostasis in the periphery.

In fact, in order to help boost immunity and mitigate the harmful effects of inactivity and social isolation stress on our immune system, it is imperative that you strive to maintain recommended exercise levels in times of increased infection rate, such as the COVID-19 pandemic.

The Physical Activity Guidelines for Americans recommend 150 to 300 minutes of moderate to vigorous intensity cardiorespiratory physical activity per week and two sessions per week of muscle strength training. This may be more challenging if you do not have access to gyms and parks and following social distancing and hygienic guidelines. There are many creative ways to stay vigorous at home nevertheless. As we have seen during the COVID-19 pandemic, increased home-based exercise, such as online instructor-led classes, are useful for some people during these stressful times. However, specialized equipment is not required; keeping active indoors or outdoors through activities such as walking and gardening can also be beneficial. This includes my personal favorite form of exercise, which is dancing.

While exercise might not prevent you from developing COVID-19, current studies of viral infections indicate that physically active people will have less severe symptoms, shorter recovery times, and may be less likely to infect others they come into contact with. Exercise is also likely to be most helpful if you are asymptomatic or experiencing only mild symptoms. In addition, exercise training has been shown to improve immune responses to both the influenza and pneumococcal vaccines.

MODERATE-TO-VIGOROUS EXERCISE

Acute exercise (moderate-to-vigorous intensity, less than 60 min) is now viewed as an important immune system support to stimulate the ongoing exchange of distinct and highly active immune cell subtypes between the circulation and tissues. In particular, each exercise routine improves the anti-pathogen activity of tissue macrophages—white blood cells—in conjunction with an increased recirculation of immunoglobulins, anti-inflammatory cytokines, neutrophils, NK cells, cytotoxic T cells, and immature B cells. These acute changes have an additive effect to enhance immune defense activity and metabolic health.

The most important finding that has emerged from exercise immunology studies is that positive immune changes take place during each bout of moderate physical activity. Over time, this translates to fewer days of sickness with the common cold and other upper respiratory tract infections. This is consistent with public health guidelines urging individuals to engage in routine physical activity of 30 minutes or more. There is a general consensus that regular bouts of short-lasting (up to 45 minutes) moderate intensity exercise is beneficial for host immune defense, particularly in older adults and people with chronic diseases.

VIGOROUS EXERCISE PROGRAM

In contrast, infection rate is reported to be higher among extreme performance athletes and is second only to injury for the number of training days lost during preparation for major events. This has shaped the common view that very vigorous exercise (for example, those activities practiced by high performance athletes/ military personnel that greatly exceed recommended physical activity guidelines) can suppress immunity and increase infection risk.

Numerous studies, over the last 35 years, report an increase in upper respiratory infection (URI) symptoms in athletes during periods of heavy training and competition. Challenges athletes face, such as heavy exercise and life stress, influence immune function. It occurs via activation of the hypothalamic-pituitary-adrenal axis—central stress response system—and the sympathetic nervous system—fight-or-flight—and the resulting immunoregulatory hormones, which regulate number and activity of white blood cells.

Both innate and acquired immunity are often reported to decrease transiently in the hours after heavy exertion, typically 15 to 70 percent. In fact, prolonged heavy training sessions have been shown to decrease immune function which may provide an opportunity for infections to take hold. Whether the observed changes in immunity with acute strenuous exercise or periods of heavy training account for the increased susceptibility to URI symptoms remains contentious. In other words, the idea that exercise can suppress immunity and increase infection risk independently of the many other factors (such as anxiety, sleep disruption, travel, exposure, nutritional deficits, and environmental extremes) experienced by these individuals has recently been a subject up for discussion. More research needs to be performed in order to examine the complex questions that surround this contentious issue in the field of exercise immunology.

How Aggressive Exercise May Harm Your Immune System

The following outlines how aggressive exercise can harm and suppress your immune system:

- Both innate and acquired immunity are often observed to decrease, typically 15 to 25 percent, in individuals that are athletes and aggressively exercise

- Decreases IL-2 after endurance exercise

- Depletes the body of important nutrients

- Elicits mobilization and functional augmentation of neutrophils and monocytes—types of white blood cells

- Endurance exercise induces systemic release of granulocyte colony-stimulating factor (G-CSF), macrophage CSF (M-CSF), IL-8 and monocyte chemotactic protein 1 (MCP-1)

- Evidence that several immune parameters are suppressed during prolonged periods of intense exercise training, which include: decreases in neutrophil function, serum and salivary immunoglobulin concentrations, natural killer cell number, and possibly cytotoxic activity in peripheral blood

- Exercise-associated depressed immune function

- Exercise-associated muscle damage

- Increases cortisol levels

- Initiation of the inflammatory cytokine cascade

- It causes oxidative stress which affects an imbalance between the systemic manifestation of reactive oxygen species (ROS) and a biological system's ability to readily detoxify the reactive intermediates or to repair the resulting damage.

- May increase testosterone levels in women

- May lower testosterone levels in males

- May produce alterations in their hypothalamic-pituitary-gonadal (HPG) axis resulting in an imbalance between the hormones

- Plasma concentrations of G-CSF, granulocyte-macrophage colony-stimulating factor, M-CSF, IL-8, and MCP-1—normally low, stimulates bone marrow to produce white blood cells and stems cell to be released into the bloodstream—is increased immediately after short-duration exercise

- Promotes poor sleep hygiene

- Sets up an inflammatory response

- Studies have shown the incidence of symptoms of upper respiratory tract infection increases during periods of endurance training.

- Temporary immunosuppression

- Transient immune dysfunction by decreasing immune cell metabolic capacity

The good news is that the small changes of these pro-inflammatory and immunomodulatory cytokines could well be mediated by anti-inflammatory cytokines, such as IL-1 receptor antagonist (IL-1ra), IL-6 and IL-10 and cytokine inhibitors (cortisol, prostaglandin E2 and soluble receptors against TNF and IL-2), which are known to increase markedly in the circulation following endurance exercise. More research needs to be done in this area.

How Aggressive Exercise
May Positively Affect Your Immune System

Since exercise increases blood flow as your muscles contract, it also increases the of circulation of immune cells. In cranking up your circulation, it has been found to:

- Reduce stress

- Have drug-like effects that may alter the cross-talk unwanted signals between the immune system and tumorigenesis—formation of tumors. For example, exercise may increase intra-tumoral cytotoxic T cell infiltration and reduce regulatory T cell infiltration, enhance the recirculation and function of tumor-specific NK cells, and decrease inflammatory influences that support cancer cell growth.

- Help regulate blood sugar to keep you young

As you have seen, the risk of upper respiratory tract infections can increase when athletes push beyond normal limits. These immune changes occur in several compartments of the immune system and body. During this "open window" of impaired immunity (between 3 and 72 hours, depending on the immune measure), viruses and bacteria may gain a foothold, increasing the risk of subclinical and clinical infection.

NUTRITIONAL REPLENISHMENT FOR VIGOROUS EXERCISE

The risk of infection is increased if the individual's nutritional status is not optimal, particularly if heavy exertion lasts longer than 90 minutes. Vigorous exercise depletes the body of important nutrients, such as coenzyme Q-10 and alpha lipoic acid.

COENZYME Q-10

Coenzyme Q-10 (Co Q-10), also known as ubiquinone, is a fat-soluble nutrient that is made in nearly all of the body's tissues. Coenzyme Q-10 is one of the fueling sources of the body, since it boosts mitochondrial function and plays a vital role in the electron transport chain facilitating the transfer of electrons into ATP—energy carrying molecule in cells. Furthermore, coenzyme Q-10 is a free radical scavenger reducing oxidative damage. The body makes less Co Q-10 with age, starting at about age 50.

■ Functions of Coenzyme Q-10

- Enhances the regeneration of vitamin E
- Is a coenzyme in energy-producing metabolic pathways
- Is an antioxidant
- Is heart protective
- Lowers blood pressure
- Neuroprotective
- Positive effects on endothelial function (regulating inflammation in the tissues)
- Reduces platelet stickiness
- Regulates genomic expression
- Stimulates the immune system

■ Causes of Coenzyme Q-10 Deficiency

- Aging process
- Deficiency of vitamins B1, B5, B5, folate, and B12
- Excessive exercise
- Genetic mutations/genetic defects
- Hyperthyroidism (over-production of thyroid hormone)
- Malabsorption due to celiac disease or sprue
- Malabsorption due to steatorrhea (excessive fat in stools)
- Malabsorption due to surgery
- Medicines and over-the-counter supplements that are usually used for weight loss to decrease fat absorption
- Taurine deficiency

- Medications, such as the ones below, are a major cause of Q-10 deficiency:
  - Adriamycin
  - Beta blockers
  - Chlorpromazine
  - Clonidine
  - Desipramine
  - Doxepin
  - Fluphenazine
  - Gemfibrozil
  - Glucophage
  - Glyburide
  - Haloperidol
  - Hydralazine
  - Hydrochlorothiazide
  - Imipramine
  - Phenothiazines
  - Protriptyline
  - Statin drugs
  - Tolazamide
  - Trimipramine

■ Recommended Daily Dosage

Depending on your age, level of exercise, and medications you may be taking, take 100 to 400 milligrams daily. Do not use if pregnant or if you are breast feeding. If you are over the age of 50, 100 mg a day is great dosage to start with. If you are taking a blood thinner, consult your doctor before using.

■ Side Effects and Contraindications

The following side effects can occur from taking CoQ_{10} supplementation. However, they are usually less severe if you take the supplement after meals.

- Abdominal discomfort
- Appetite loss
- Diarrhea (when doses taken are greater than 100 milligrams)
- Heartburn
- Increase in liver enzymes (when doses taken are greater than 300 milligrams)
- Insomnia (when doses taken are greater than 100 milligrams)
- Irritability
- Palpitations
- Photophobia

ALPHA LIPOIC ACID

Alpha-lipoic acid is a nutrient that is both fat and water soluble. It is an antioxidant that is made by the body and helps turn glucose into energy. Unfortunately, the body makes less alpha-lipoic acid as you age.

■ Functions of Alpha Lipoic Acid

- Acts as a metal chelator for cadmium, copper, and iron
- Helps prevent cataracts
- Improves endothelial function (which helps prevent heart disease)
- Improves the immune system
- Increases glutathione by 30 percent to 70 percent
- Increases nitric oxide synthesis
- Is a cofactor for mitochondrial enzymes, which are needed for energy production

- Liver protective
- Lowers blood pressure
- Lowers levels of calcium if elevated
- Modulates gene expression to help insulin work more effectively in the body
- Neuroprotective
- Neutralizes free radical, since it is an antioxidant
- Promotes glucose uptake and utilization
- Protects collagen in the skin from cross-linking, which can cause sagging and wrinkles
- Recycles coenzyme Q-10, glutathione, vitamins C and E
- Slows brain aging
- Stimulates the sprouting of new nerve fibers on nerve cells.
- Stops activation of NF-kappa B (a protein complex. If activated, it can increase your risk of developing cancer, heart disease, and other illnesses) in your cells
- Stops adhesion of macrophages (large white blood cells that can cause heart disease) to your arterial wall

Causes of Deficiency

- Aging process
- Nutritional deficiencies

Signs and Symptoms of Deficiency

- Cataracts
- Cognitive decline
- Fatigue
- Insulin resistance/diabetes
- Skin wrinkling

Recommended Daily Dosage

Take 50 to 400 milligrams daily.

Side Effects and Contraindications

If you take 600 mg a day or more of alpha lipoic acid, you may experience decreased conversion of T4 to T3, and you may have resultant symptoms of hypothyroidism (low thyroid function). For some conditions you may need high dose alpha lipoic acid, such as hepatitis C. Do not use a dose of about 500 mg a day unless you are under the direction of a healthcare provider that can monitor your thyroid studies on a regular basis.

Other possible side effects include the following (more common at doses above 1,200 mg a day): fatigue, insomnia, diarrhea, skin rash, nausea, vomiting, headaches, and itching sensations.

If you are using insulin or an oral hypoglycemic agent along with alpha lipoic acid, then the dose of insulin or oral hypoglycemic agent may need to be lowered. Check your blood sugar on a regular basis.

EXERCISE INFLUENCES IMMUNOSENESCENCE

The aging process also affects how well the immune system functions. Getting older is associated with a decrease in the normal functioning of the immune system, which is called "immunosenescence." This condition contributes to poorer vaccine responses, increased incidence of infection, and malignancy seen in older individuals. However, regular exercise is capable of policing the immune system and delaying the onset of immunosenescence.

Consistent exercise has been associated with the following mechanisms that enhance the immune system for older adults:

- Balances levels of sex hormones in women

- Boosts the function of natural killer cells
  - CD4:CD8 ratio <1.0 (blood tests to monitor the immune system if you have AIDS)

- Enhanced vaccination responses
  - High numbers and proportions of late-stage differentiated effector memory cells

- Improves lymphocyte immune surveillance by improving the transient lymphocytosis and subsequent lymphocytopenia
  - Includes low numbers and proportions of naive cells (T and B cells before they mature)

- Increased neutrophil phagocytic activity (removal of bacterial and fungal pathogens)

- Moderate exercise lowers levels of inflammatory cytokines, which decreases the risk of developing diseases such as heart disease, type 2 diabetes, osteoporosis, Alzheimer's disease, and even cancer.

Increased T cell proliferative capacity aids the following processes that are part of immunosenescence:

- Increases level of testosterone in males

- Induces activity of the growth hormone-insulin-like growth factor-1 axis and therefore produces positive effects on skeletal muscle

- Longer leukocyte telomere lengths (associated with life span)

- Lowers circulatory levels of inflammatory cytokines

- Lowers numbers of exhausted/senescent T cells (depletion of effector T cells)

- Lowers inflammatory response to bacterial challenge

- Poor proliferative responses to mitogens—cell division

Therefore, exercise can improve the immune system in individuals over the age of 65, which are a group of people where the immune system has shown a significant decline due to the aging process. This same population has also been hard hurt by recent viral infections, such as COVID-19.

EXERCISE AND THE GUT MICROBIOTA

Last, a new area of study involves the fact that exercise diversifies the gut microbiota. The gastrointestinal tract is colonized by trillions of microorganisms that include a gene set much greater than of the human genome. The most abundant bacterial phyla are the Firmicutes (about 60 percent) and the Bacteriodetes (about 20 percent), with low proportions of Actinobacteria, Proteobacteria, and Verrucomicrobia. One-third of the adult gut microbiota is similar between most individuals, but diversity is associated with a healthier status.

Your gut bacteria composition and diversity are influenced by a variety of factors, including dietary and exercise habits, age, genetics, ethnicity, antibiotics, health, and disease. Even weight affects this relationship. In a medical trial, beta diversity analysis revealed that exercise-induced alterations of the gut microbiota were dependent on obesity status. Exercise increased fecal concentrations of short-chain fatty acids in lean, but not obese, participants. In addition, the study found that exercise-induced changes in the microbiota were largely reversed once exercise training ceased. These findings suggest that exercise training induces compositional and functional changes in the human gut microbiota that are dependent on obesity status, independent of diet, and contingent on the sustainment of exercise.

Furthermore, exercise is a modulator of intestinal microbiome composition since it is associated with increased biodiversity—diversity of microbes in the gut—and beneficial metabolic functions. Moreover, your gut microbiota can influence the pathophysiology—functional changes—of several distant organs, including the skeletal muscle. In addition, a gut muscle axis, in which our gut microbiota are linked with muscle function and metabolism, may in fact regulate muscle protein deposition and muscle function. In older individuals, this axis may be involved in the pathogenesis of muscle wasting disorders through multiple mechanisms, involving transfer of stimuli from dietary nutrients, modulation of inflammation, and even insulin sensitivity—describes how sensitive the body's effects are to the hormone insulin. The immune system plays a fundamental role in these processes, being influenced by microbiome composition and at the same time contributing to the fundamental process of cellular growth.

Likewise, the gut microbiome and its influence on host behavior, intestinal barrier and immune function are believed to be a critical aspect of the brain-gut axis. Recent evidence in the animal model reveals that there is a high correlation between physical and emotional stress during exercise and changes in gastrointestinal microbiota composition. In addition, diet dramatically modulates the composition of the gut microbiota since the gut microbiota influences human health and immune function, in part through the fermentation of indigestible food components in the large intestine. Consequently, the microbiome and derived metabolites—necessary for metabolism—including short chain fatty acids and bio-transformed bile acids, have been shown to influence immune function both within the gut and throughout the remainder of the body.

Preliminary results obtained from studies using probiotics and prebiotics show that the microbiota acts like an endocrine organ by secreting serotonin, dopamine, or other neurotransmitters, and may control the HPA axis in athletes and individuals that exercise daily. Current dietary recommendations for elite athletes are primarily based on a low consumption of plant polysaccharides, which is associated with reduced microbiota diversity and functionality producing less short chain fatty acids and neurotransmitters. It really is all about balance. Training to exhaustion can be associated with dysbiosis (microbial imbalance or malabsorption) of the intestinal microbiome, promoting inflammation and negative metabolic consequences. For a longer discussion of this subject, see the chapter 7 on GI Health and the Immune system in this book.

CONCLUSION

As you have seen in this chapter, there are many ways to improve your immune system, however moderation is the key to health. Too little exercise or too vigorous an exercise program can compromise the immune system. A planned, well-thought out, moderate exercise program is one of the main recipes to building and enhancing your immune system, Several epidemiologic studies suggest that regular physical activity is associated with decreased mortality and incidence rates for influenza and pneumonia.

In addition, exercise may help rejuvenate the aging immune system by delaying the onset of immunological aging or even rejuvenating aged immune profiles. There is also increasing evidence that exercise training has a summation effect over time in modulating tumor growth, atherosclerosis, and other disease processes along with immune building.

7

Your Gut
A Healthy Gut Equals
a Healthy Immune System

You are what you eat! Triggers, such as a poor diet, can lead to gastrointestinal (GI) challenges, and gastrointestinal imbalances, which have been identified as a factor in many immune and autoimmune conditions. Recent research certainly supports this statement. Growing evidence also supports the concept that the microbiota plays a significant role in maintaining nutritional, metabolic, and immunologic homeostasis in the host. In addition, the microbiota, not only maintains gastrointestinal homeostasis but also exerts metabolic functions in nutrient digestion and absorption, detoxification, and vitamin production.

As you review this chapter it is important to understand two terms which sometimes are used interchangeable, however they do not really mean the same thing. Human **microbiota** is the term used to describe all the microorganisms (bacteria, eukaryotes, archaea, and viruses) within the human body; in other words, the community of microorganisms themselves. The **microbiome** is defined as the complete catalog of these microbes and their genes; in other words, the collective genomes of the micro-organisms in a particular environment.

This chapter explores metabolic approaches to gastrointestinal (GI) imbalance. The regulatory control of digestion and absorption are under strict management of the neuronal and hormonal systems, and there are many causes of digestion and absorption problems. Some are due to mechanical issues, such as mastication, motility, and permeability. Likewise, many times GI complaints are due to multifactorial dysfunctions. Inability to digest effectively may lead to bloating, gas indigestion, constipation, diarrhea, or abdominal complaints.

Abnormal permeability of the intestinal wall can lead to leaky gut syndrome, yeast overgrowth, development of food allergies, and toxin production. Low gastric acidity can lead to symptoms of bloating, belching, burning, and flatulence immediately after ingesting a meal. A deficiency of gastric enzymes may lead to delayed breakdown of protein and result in symptoms of protein maldigestion. Likewise, pancreatic enzymes are required to break proteins into peptides, and a deficiency of proteolytic enzymes (produced by the pancreas and stomach) is another reason that the digestion of protein by the body may not work optimally.

Therapeutic approaches to restoration of enzymatic function and to reduce inflammation are key components that are addressed in this section, along with the chapter on inflammation. Food triggers, such as allergies to gluten and dairy, will also be examined. You will learn how to optimize the health of your gut through the "5 R" program of remove, replace, repopulate, repair, and rebalance.

THE GASTROINTESTINAL TRACT

Your gastrointestinal tract (GI tract) is literally 70 percent of your immune system. In the GI tract is the largest blood supply in the body using 1/3 of the total blood flow from the heart. The gut flora contain 400 different microbial species which include the following: Bacteroides, *Lactobacillus*, Clostridum, Fusobacterium, Bifidobacterium, Eubacterium, Peptococcus, Peptostreptoccus, Escherichia, and Vellonella along with many others.

In fact, the numbers of bacterial and human cells are estimated to be—close to—or equal to each other: about 3.9×10^{13} bacterial cells and 3.0×10^{13} human cells. To be more specific, about 100 trillion micro-organisms (most of them bacteria, but also viruses, fungi, and protozoa) exist in the human gastrointestinal tract. Consequently, the gut has a massive amount of influence on your metabolism. It is really the hidden organ! It has greater metabolic activity than the liver, with 10 times the number of cells and 100 times the genomic material. The cells of the intestinal tract are shed and replaced every 3 to 6 days. Therefore, they are very sensitive to nutrition and lifestyle choices.

Function of the GI Tract

Therefore, if your gut is not healthy you are not healthy. Dr. Jill Carnahan is one of the gurus in the world concerning GI health. She states the following: "You are what you eat, and then absorb, and then what you do or do not detoxify." What does the GI tract actually do in the body? The following are the major functions of the GI tract:

Digestion. This is the process whereby our food is broken down into smaller portions that are more easily absorbed by the intestines.

Absorption. This is the process whereby the digested food is taken up by the intestine and delivered to the body for utilization as energy, nutrition, and other cellular functions.

Detoxification. This is the complex process involving the liver and GI tract whereby toxins are metabolized for elimination from the body. Toxins include such things as medication we take that must be metabolized, to pesticides, preservatives, dyes, and flavor-enhancers we ingest knowingly in our food, as well as the over 4 million chemicals present in our environment not intended for use in our bodies.

Elimination. After digestion has occurred, and the metabolic phase of detoxification is complete, the GI tract must then eliminate the digestive and metabolic wastes of these processes. Some refer to this as excretion. Transit time in the intestine from mouth to rectum should be 24 to 30 hours. In the U.S. it is about 48 hours.

Exclusion. This refers to the barrier function performed by the GI tract as it appropriately excludes substances from entering the body.

GI Microbiome and the GI Barrier

How do you have a healthy gut? From a traditional medicine viewpoint, you have a healthy GI tract when you have met these five major criteria: effective digestion and absorption of food, absence of GI illness, normal and stable intestinal microbiota, effective immune status, and status of well-being. There is now ample evidence that two functional entities are key to achieving and maintaining gut health. These entities are the GI microbiome and the GI barrier, which is not just a mechanical barrier assessed by permeability measurements.

Multiple functions of the GI microbiome have been described in the medical literature. The GI microbiome prevents colonization by potentially pathogenic microorganisms, provides energy for the gut wall from undigested food and it regulates the mucosal immune system. Most importantly, the GI microbiota contributes to the maintenance of an intact GI barrier, which is closely related to infectious, inflammatory, and allergic diseases.

The *gastrointestinal mucosa*—membrane rich in mucous—forms a barrier between the body and potential hostile microorganisms and toxins. In addition, the GI barrier allows the stomach to safely store the gastric acid that is necessary for digestion.

INTESTINAL DYSFUNCTION

Almost half of the adults in the U.S. experience intestinal illness at some time in their lives. Even emotional trauma can negatively impact your digestion. Dr. D.L. Berkson wrote the number one best-selling book of all time on GI health, *Healthy Digestion The Natural Way*. Much of what I have learned concerning GI health I have learned from Dr. Berkson. She is a major authority in this field. The following are signs of poor digestion and then optimal digestion—it may surprise you that to have perfect digestion, you need to have two normal bowel movements a day.

Signs of Poor Digestion

- Chronic indigestion after eating
- Chronically coated tongue
- Depressed without a reason
- Feel better if you do not eat
- Feeling stress without a cause
- Foul smelling stools
- Frequent burping, passing gas, and/or bloated stomach
- Frequently cold for no reason
- Increase in pulse of 20 to 25 beats within 15 minutes after eating
- Less than one bowel movement a day
- Need to loosen your belt after eating even though you did not overeat
- Poor sleeping habits/waking up tired
- Undigested food in stools

Signs of Optimal Digestion

- Do not have frequent mood swings, shakiness, anxiety, or depression without a reason
- Feel better after exercising
- Feel good after eating and several hours later
- Good energy level throughout the day
- No extreme food cravings
- No undigested food in stools
- Sleep well and wake up rested
- Stools do not smell
- Two bowel movements a day
- Warm extremities

The GI tract needs basic nutrients; B vitamins, such as B1, B6, and folic acid, and also vitamins A, C, D, and E. The gut also needs minerals, such as zinc, selenium, manganese, molybdenum, magnesium, and the amino acid arginine. Therefore, starting with a good multivitamin that is pharmaceutical grade is a great place to start your journey to optimal GI health.

DYSBIOSIS

Dysbiosis is an inflammatory disease of the GI tract due to imbalance of intestinal bacteria. Consequences of dysbiosis are great, including loss of good bacteria and loss of the production of some important vitamins. In addition, the gastrointestinal tract is one of the body's five organs of detoxification. Consequently, if you have dysbiosis, your body does not detoxify well. Furthermore, if you have dysbiosis you lose protection from chemical toxins and antibiotics along with having a subsequent overgrowth of harmful bacteria.

■ Symptoms of Dysbiosis

Many symptoms can occur due to dysbiosis, including ones that are related to both inside and outside the GI tract, extra-intestinal symptoms, which Dr. Berkson brilliantly discusses in her book.

Common symptoms include:

- Abdominal distention and bloating
- Abdominal pain
- Altered bowel function (constipation and/or diarrhea)
- Belching
- Bloating
- Cramping

- Cramps and spasms
- Flatulence
- Halitosis
- Heartburn
- Hypersecretion of colonic mucus
- Nausea

Extra-intestinal symptoms linked to dysbiosis include:

- Anxiety
- Arthralgias
- Brain fog
- Cognitive and memory deficit
- Depression
- Fatigue
- Fever of unknown origin
- Frequent urination

- Malaise
- Myalgias
- Palpitations
- Phlebitis
- Pruritis
- Seizures
- Skin rashes
- Vasculitis

Causes of Dysbiosis

The etiologies of dysbiosis are numerous. Consequently, it is a common problem. It is often due to one or a combination of the following:

- Alcohol abuse
  - Ethanol and acetaldehyde (one of the breakdown products of ethanol) disrupt the tight junctions in the cells lining the intestines which increases membrane permeability.
- Alcohol consumption
- Artificial sweeteners cause glucose intolerance by altering the gut microbiota and induce dysbiosis
- Carbohydrate malabsorption
  - Consumption of infected foods
- Corticosteroid use
- Diminished bile
- Excessive stress
- Food allergies and sensitivities
- Free radical production
- Gastrointestinal surgeries
- Hypoxia/exposure to extreme altitude
- Immune deficiencies
- Improper fasting or dieting
- Lectins are protein fragments of foods that are not completely digested that bind with specific sugars on the surface cells throughout the body. They stick to the lining of the GI tract, which causes inflammation and can destroy cell membranes. Lectins flatten the intestinal villi and consequently decrease the absorption of nutrients.
- Low levels of hydrochloric acid in the stomach
- Nutritional deficiencies
- Pancreatic insufficiency
- Repeated use of antibiotics
- Travel
- Use of non-steroidal anti-inflammatory drugs (NSAIDs)

- Damage the mucosal lining
- Damage the mitochondria (turn energy from food into energy the cell can use)
- Breakdown intercellular integrity
- Recirculate waste products from the liver
- Activate neutrophils caused by the escape of bacteria and large molecules of undigested food through the compromised intestinal barrier
- Viruses like rotaviruses have proteins on their outer surfaces that can open the cellular spaces between the tight junctions of the GI mucous cells
- Yeast infections

SMALL INTESTINAL BOWEL OVERGROWTH (SIBO)

As previous mentioned, the human intestinal microbiota is composed of trillions of cells, including bacteria, viruses, and fungi and it creates a complex polymicrobial ecology—a presence of several species. This is characterized by its high population density as well as wide diversity and complexity of interaction. An imbalance of this complex intestinal microbiome, both qualitative and quantitative, may have serious health consequence for the body, including small intestinal bowel overgrowth, commonly called SIBO. It is a specific kind of dysbiosis.

In other words, the GI tract is full of bacteria, it just had to be the right kind of bacteria and the right number of bacteria. SIBO is defined as an increase in the number and/or alteration in the type of bacteria in the upper gastrointestinal tract where it does not belong. This overgrowth of bacteria usually only occurs in the colon which is the large intestine. The body has mechanisms for preventing bacterial overgrowth: gastric acid secretion, intestinal motility, intact ileocecal valve, immunoglobulins within intestinal secretion, and bacteriostatic properties of pancreatic and biliary secretion. In some people more than one cause may be involved in the development of SIBO.

■ Symptoms

Symptoms related to SIBO are:

- Abdominal pain
- Bloating
- Diarrhea
- Malabsorption
- Malnutrition
- Weight loss

The diagnosis is made by an upper GI aspirate or 3-hour lactulose breath test for hydrogen/methane.

■ Causes

SIBO is commonly the cause of a (motility) movement problem in the small intestine. If something impairs the movement, such as one or more of the following, the small intestine can't eliminate the bacteria.

- Achlorhydria (low stomach acid)
- Excessive use of antibiotics
- Gastrointestinal conditions (irritable bowel syndrome, inflammatory bowel disease, and celiac disease)
- History of bowel surgeries or anatomical abnormalities (small intestinal obstruction, diverticula, fistulae, surgical blind loop, previous ileocecal resections)
- Immunodeficiency syndromes
- Impaired valve separating the small and large intestines (ileocecal valve)
- Long-term use of proton pump inhibitors (PPIs)
- Motility disorders (scleroderma, autonomic neuropathy in diabetes mellitus, post-radiation enteropathy, small intestinal pseudo-obstruction)
- Pancreatic exocrine insufficiency
- Poor gallbladder function
- Poor nutrient status (deficiencies of choline, taurine, magnesium and others)

■ Therapies

Small intestinal bowel overgrowth therapies are designed to correct the balance of bacteria in the small intestines. Doctors begin treating SIBO by examining the cause of the underlying disease. Nutritional therapies and even antibiotics are also commonly required.

■ Medications

Therapies for SIBO may include medications such as:

Rifaximin is an antibiotic that fights a bacterial infection only in the intestine. If you are a methane producer your doctor may add metronidazole or neomycin. Low dose erythromycin may be useful.

Prokinetic medications are also commonly prescribed which enhance GI motility by increasing the frequency or strength of contractions.

Low dose naltrexone is a novel anti-inflammatory agent with promising immunomodulatory affects. (*See* chapter on inflammation for more information.)

■ Herbal Therapies

These therapies, for one to two months, are also commonly employed, such as:

Berberine: 500 mg three times a day

Oregano: 200 mg three times a day

Garlic extract: 450 mg twice a day

Iberogast: a mixture of nine medicinal plant extracts:

- Angelica root (Angelicae radix)
- Balm leaf (Melissae folium)
- Bitter candytuft (Iberis amara)
- Caraway fruit (Carvi fructus)
- Celandine herb (Chelidonium majus)
- Chamomile flower (Matricariae flos)
- Liquorice root (Liquiritiae radix)
- Milk thistle fruit (Silybi mariani fructus)
- Peppermint herb (Menthae piperitae folium)

Iberogast, as described above, is also effective. Furthermore, ginger has been shown to be beneficial.

■ Probiotics

Initially probiotics may be contraindicated because SIBO often involves an overgrowth of D-lactate-producing bacteria. Therefore, probiotics may be added a couple of weeks later. It is important not to eat 2 hours before bedtime and to have 4 to 5 hours between meals.

■ Diet

A SIBO diet should consist of foods high in fiber and low in sugar. Some foods contain low quantities of FODMAPs (carbohydrates—sugars—that the small intestine absorbs poorly) in small servings but should be curbed because larger servings would increase the FODMAPs. FODMAP represents fermentable oligosaccharides, disaccharides, monosaccharides and polyols.

Low FODMAPs Diet

A low FODMAP diet is part of the current therapy for SIBO which is effective in many patients:

Dairy/alternatives. Almond milk, coconut milk, hemp milk, rice milk, butter, hard or aged cheese (cheddar, parmesan, brie)

Fruits. Bananas (unripe,) berries, cantaloupe, avocado, grapes, honeydew, olives, papaya, pineapple, rhubarb

Grains. Amaranth, brown rice, bulgur wheat, oats, gluten-free products, quinoa

Nuts, legumes, seeds. Almonds. hazelnuts, macadamia nuts pecan, walnuts, chia seeds, pumpkin seeds, sesame seeds, sunflower seeds

Vegetables. Arugula, broccoli, carrots, cabbage, corn, eggplant, kale, parsnip, spinach, sweet potatoes, tomatoes, turnips, zucchini

High FODMAPs Diet

Foods high in FODMAPs are beneficial for most people because of their nutritional content. However, if you have SIBO or irritable bowel syndrome (IBS) foods that are high in FODMAPs can disrupt your digestive tract and can cause abdominal pain, gas, and bloating. Therefore, if you have SIBO or IBS avoid the following foods.

Dairy. Cow's milk, buttermilk, cream, ice cream, margarine, soft cheeses (cottage cheese, ricotta) soy milk, yogurt

Food additives. Chicory root and xylitol. Inulin should be initially avoided but may be added into the diet from a natural source after a couple of weeks.

Fruits. Ripe bananas, raspberries, cherries, pears, apples, mango, nectarines, peaches, pears, pomegranate, watermelon, canned/dried fruit

Grains. Barley, couscous, farro (high-fiber, high protein whole grain), rye, semolina, wheat

Nuts, legumes, seeds. Baked beans, black-eyed peas, butter beans, chickpeas, lentils, kidney beans, lima beans, soybeans, split peas

Sweeteners. Honey, agave nectar

Vegetables. Artichokes, asparagus, beets, Brussel sprouts, cabbage, garlic, mushrooms, okra, peas, snow peas, sugar snap peas

Inulins

Inulins are a type of polysaccharide found inside many varieties of plants used to store energy. They also belong to a type of dietary fiber known as fructans. Fructans are part of the oligosaccharides group in the FODMAP acronym and can cause serious digestive symptoms for individuals with irritable bowel syndrome and other digestive disorders. This is due to inulin not being absorbed in the small intestine, which means when it reaches the large intestine it is devoured by the gut bacteria. This fermentation can cause bloating, abdominal pain, wind, and loose stools.

Why is inulin consumption recommended for some people?

Inulin can function as a prebiotic, which means it feeds good bacteria. Inulin as a prebiotic has the following functions:

- Supports the immune system

- Increases the amount of calcium and minerals being absorbed by the body

- Improves intestinal complaints as long as it does not cause a FODMAP reaction

- Decreases constipation by increasing the amount of fiber in the diet

    Inulin occurs naturally in chicory, globe and Jerusalem artichokes, garlic, onion, barley, wheat, and ripe bananas.

■ Conditions Associated with Small Intestinal Bowel Overgrowth

SIBO is linked to many disorders, as a cause, as an effect, or as a co-existing condition. If you have had or are experiencing one of the following conditions, testing for SIBO may be beneficial.

- Achlorhydria
- Acne
- Aging process
- Bariatric surgery
- Bowel resection surgery
- Celiac disease
- Chronic antibiotic use
- Chronic pancreatitis
- Cirrhosis
- Collagen vascular disease
- Crohn's disease
- Dysmotility
- Fibromyalgia
- Hypochlorhydria

- IgA deficiency
- Immune deficiency
- Malnutrition
- Non-alcoholic steatorrhea (excessive fat in feces)

- Protein pump inhibitor use
- Rosacea
- Short bowel syndrome

SMALL INTESTINAL FUNGAL OVERGROWTH

Small intestinal fungal overgrowth (SIFO) is characterized by the presence of excessive amounts of fungus in the small intestine. It has been known for years that candidiasis (yeast infections) can cause symptoms in the GI tract of patients that are immunocompromised. Now in the medical literature, studies are revealing that SIFO can cause symptoms in patients that are otherwise healthy. Symptoms of SIFO are quite varied.

■ Symptoms and Signs

The signs and symptoms of SIFO are consistent with other conditions that cause chronic or recurring GI symptoms. Several of the most common symptoms include:

- Belching
- Bloating
- Depression
- Diarrhea
- Fatigue

- Gas
- Indigestion
- Migraines
- Nausea

■ Causes

The two main causes that are known for SIFO are intestinal dysmotility and reduced amounts of stomach acid due to the use of proton pump inhibitors.

Intestinal dysmotility: When the contractions of the intestinal smooth muscle are impaired it can cause digestive disorders, If the contractions are slowed down and less frequent, they can cause constipation; if they are sped up and more frequent, it can cause loose stools or diarrhea.

Proton pump inhibitors: PPI or proton pump inhibitors reduce the production of acid and lower levels of acid in the stomach. PPI's are used as a treatment for GERD, stomach ulcers, and erosive esophagitis, however the reduction of the stomach acid in the stomach may lead to SIFO.

In addition, if you have gone through antibiotic therapy recently or dental work, if you consume a diet high in simple carbohydrates and experience recurring vaginal yeast or chronic sinusitis, you may be prone to an increased risk of developing SIFO.

LEAKY GUT SYNDROME

If you have dysbiosis, including SIBO, this commonly leads to leaky gut syndrome. Leaky gut syndrome occurs when there is damage to the lining of the bowel which results in increased permeability. Intestinal permeability is a term describing the control of material passing from inside the gastrointestinal tract through the cells lining the gut wall into the remainder of the body.

The intestine normally exhibits some permeability, which allows nutrients to pass through the gut, while also maintaining a barrier function to keep potentially harmful substances from leaving the intestine and moving to the remainder of the body. Increased permeability allows toxins to re-enter the blood stream and also if you are taking medication, to possibly get the medication a second time.

■ Symptoms and Signs

Symptoms and signs of a leaky gut may include:

- Abdominal pain
- Aches and pain in joints
- Aggressive behavior
- Anxiety
- Asthma
- Bed-wetting
- Bladder infections
- Bloating
- Chronic fatigue
- Chronic joint pain
- Confusion
- Constipation
- Cramps
- Diarrhea
- Exercise intolerance
- Fatigue
- Fever of unknown cause
- Foggy thinking
- Food sensitivities
- Gas
- Indigestion
- Inflammatory skin conditions
- Learning disorders
- Mood swings
- Muscle pains
- Nervousness

- PMS
- Recurring infections

- Shortness of breath
- Skin rash

■ Causes of Increased Intestinal Permeability

There is no single cause for leaky gut syndrome, but there are several feasible reasons for its development. Some of the underlying causes of leaky gut include:

- Aging process
- Celiac disease
- Chronic alcoholism
- Diarrhea
- Food allergies
- Inflammatory bowel disease
- NSAIDs drugs

- Nutritional depletions
- Protozoal infections
- Small intestinal bacterial overgrowth (SIBO)
- Strenuous exercise
- Stress
- Toxic exposure

■ Conditions Associated With Leaky Gut Syndrome

Multiple diseases may emerge or be amplified due to a leaky gut, and they may extend beyond the gastro-intestinal tract. The following are common:

- Acne
- Aging
- AIDS
- Alcoholism
- Allergies/food sensitivities
- Ankylosing spondylitis
- Arthritis
- Asthma
- Autism
- Burns
- Candida infections
- Celiac disease
- Chemical sensitivities

- Chemotherapy
- Chronic fatigue syndrome
- Crohn's disease
- Cystic fibrosis
- Eczema
- Environmental illness
- Fibromyalgia
- Hyperactivity
- IBS
- Intestinal infections
- Liver dysfunction
- Lupus
- Malabsorption

- Malnutrition
- Psoriasis
- Reiter's syndrome
- Rheumatoid arthritis

- Schizophrenia
- Trauma
- Ulcerative colitis

Many people have a GI tract that is not healthy due to all the reasons previously discussed. The good news is that the 5 R program for gut restoration is able to help almost all individuals have a healthy gut, which produces a healthy immune system.

THE 5 R PROGRAM FOR GUT RESTORATION

The 5 R program for gut restoration was developed by the Institute For Functional Medicine. It is a complete and comprehensive approach that not only improves symptoms, but it helps heal with long-lasting results. The aim of the program is to address dietary changes, to normalize digestion and absorption, to balance gastrointestinal bacteria, to create a balanced system of detoxification, and to promote healing of the gut.

The following five key points are involved in the 5 R program: remove, replace, repopulate, repair, and rebalance. A comprehensive 5 R program takes roughly about 3 to 6 months to complete. It is essential that you are amenable to implement the challenging dietary changes of the program, as without the dietary portion you cannot attain the maximum therapeutic benefit.

Therefore, it is crucial to start the gut restoration program by eating a healthy diet. One study showed that your diet has the most powerful influence on gut microbial communities, more than anything else that can be done if you are basically healthy to begin with.

1. REMOVE

The first step in helping to achieve optimal GI health is to remove anything that has a negative impact on the gut. Finding a trigger may not be initially obvious and therefore may take some time. Triggers may include the following:

Food allergies. Food allergies or sensitivities are a common item. At least 60 percent of Americans have food allergies. It may take a while to discover some food sensitivities, since symptoms may not occur until hours or days later. An allergy elimination diet is one method of evaluating foods you may have a sensitivity to. They may include gut irritants, such as alcohol, caffeine, processed food, and food additives. Also, food allergy testing that examines both allergies that are IgG and IgE related may be beneficial to have performed.

Pathogens. Pathogens are organisms that are not desirable, such as yeast, parasites, or pathogenic bacteria. You may need to take medication, such as antibiotics, anti-parasitic agents, or antifungal drugs. Herbal therapies may also be beneficial but commonly require six months of therapy to be effective.

Stress. Both physical and mental stress can negatively impact GI health. Changes that may occur include food cravings and appetite, alterations in gut function, and modifications to intestinal permeability.

Medications and supplements, Medications and supplements can cause gut dysfunction. The most common medications are non-steroidal anti-inflammatory drugs (NSAIDs).

Environment. Environmental stressors that are toxins in the environment can contribute to the toxic load carried by the body and have a negative impact on the GI tract.

Inflammation. Systemic inflammation increases intestinal permeability. A further discussion on this subject is in the last chapter of this section of the book.

2. REPLACE

Once the offending agents are removed, the next step is to replace digestive secretions that are low or lacking in your body. You may be deficient in a number of elements that are fundamental to digestion, such as stomach acid, bile, and digestive enzymes. You also may be lacking in certain nutrients. The following are digestive factors that may be important and may need replacing.

DIGESTIVE ENZYMES DEFICIENCY

Digestion decreases with age because digestive enzyme production declines which slows down or inhibits your ability to process nutrients. This may also occur if you do not chew your food well. Studies have shown that you should chew each bite of food 20 times for adequate digestion and production of digestive enzymes. Digestive enzymes have many functions in the body. They enhance digestive health, reduce autoimmunity, decrease post-surgery recover time by decreasing the need for pain relievers, and reduce swelling.

In fact, in Europe, digestive enzymes are used to treat arthritis due to their anti-inflammatory effect.

Pancreatic Enzyme Deficiency

An increase in meat and vegetable fibers in your stool suggests impaired digestion due to insufficient pancreatic enzymes or low HCL levels. There are many signs and symptoms of pancreatic enzyme deficiency:

- Fat soluble vitamin deficiencies
- Food intolerances
- Gastroesophageal reflux
- Hypochlorhydria (low stomach acid)
- Loose or watery stools
- No improvement in health when eating a good diet and taking supplements
- Post-prandial bloating, pain, or nausea ½ hour to several hours after eating (low stomach acid produces pain immediately after eating)
- Undigested food in stool

Evaluating Pancreatic Insufficiency

Measuring pancreatic elastase (PE) levels are a method of evaluating pancreatic insufficiency. PE is a proteolytic enzyme secreted exclusively by the human pancreas. It reflects overall enzyme production (amylase, lipase, and protease) and is not affected by gut transit time, not enzymatically degraded, and not affected by digestive enzyme supplementation.

- Healthy patients: PE1 >500 mcg/g
- Mild to moderate dysfunction: PE1 100-200 mcg/g
- Moderate to severe dysfunction: PE1 <100 mcg/g

Enzyme Depletion

Lifestyle choices and aging can be a factor in the body's ability to produce the needed enzymes as well as certain conditions.

- Arterial obstruction
- Bovine growth hormone used in livestock
- Celiac disease
- Cooking at high temperatures
- Fluoridation of water

- Heavy metals
- Hybridization and genetic engineering of plants
- Inflammatory disorders
- Ischemic disease
- Lactose intolerance
- Large intake of unsaturated and hydrogenated fats
- Malabsorption
- Maldigestion
- Mercury amalgam dental fillings
- Microwaving
- Pancreatic insufficiency
- Pasteurization
- Pesticides
- Radiation and electromagnetic fields
- Rheumatoid arthritis
- Root canals and hidden dental infections
- Steatorrhea (excess fat in feces)

Digestive Enzymes Replacement

Take 2 to 3 digestive enzymes just before or at the beginning of a meal. The following is an example of a common formula.

- Protease 100,000 USP units
- Lipase 20,000 USP units
- Amylase 100,000 USP units

Bitters: Bitters trigger the release of digestive enzymes in the mouth. They also increase the release of HCL in the stomach and enhance the production of bile. In addition, bitters increase the production of saliva and gastric juices which accelerates the stomach emptying causing the pancreas to release digestive enzymes. Bitter herbs have been shown to treat the following conditions: sluggish digestion, flatulence, bloating, dyspepsia, and bowel distention. An example of an excellent herbal combination of bitters is the following: ginger root, cardamom seed, centaury, astragalus root, fennel seed, rosemary leaf, and gentian root. There are also commercially formulated bitters. In addition, bitters occur in a bitter salad with dandelion leaves, escarole, endive, and other bitter salad greens which can be combined with romaine lettuce.

Enzymatic Therapy

Enzymatic therapy replacement, a medical treatment in which the enzyme level is increased, has been effective for the following conditions:

- Arterial obstruction
- Celiac disease
- Inflammatory disorders
- Ischemic disease

- Lactose intolerance
- Malabsorption
- Maldigestion
- Pancreatic insufficiency

- Rheumatoid arthritis
- Steatorrhea (excess fat in feces)
- Thrombotic disease

■ Side Effects and Contraindications

Do not take digestive enzymes if you have ulcers or any kind of active inflammatory bowel condition without consulting your healthcare provider. If the digestive enzyme contains papain do not take it if you are on the drug Coumadin, which is a blood thinner. Some digestive enzymes contain papain from papaya to assist in protein digestion. Do not use any digestive enzymes that contain papain if you are allergic to papaya.

Speak to your doctor or pharmacist to learn if any drugs you are taking might make it unwise to use digestive enzymes. Avoid enzymes with bromelain if you are allergic to pineapple, latex, wheat, celery, carrot, fennel, cypress

Types of Digestive Enzymes

There are different types of digestive enzymes which break down the food that you eat and they are produced in various areas of your body. Digestive enzymes such as:

- Amylase is produced in the mouth and it helps break down starches into simple sugars.

- Lingual lipase is secreted by the tongue to breakdown triglycerides (fats).

- Pepsin is secreted in the stomach to breakdown protein into small peptides.

- Proteolytic enzymes (other than pepsin) are released from the pancrease to further break down proteins into peptides and eventually into their components, amino acids. They are also called protease, proteinase, or peptidase.

- Pancreatic lipase is released from the pancrease to continue the breakdown of fats that began in the mouth.

- Lactase is found in the small intestine and is involved in the breakdown of lactose (milk sugar) into two simple sugars which are glucose and galactose.

pollen, or grass pollen. Furthermore, high doses of digestive enzymes can negatively impact uric acid levels. Although relatively rare, the side effects of digestive enzymes can also include the following:

- Constipation
- Cough
- Diarrhea
- Gas

- Heartburn
- Nausea
- Sore throat
- Upset stomach

GASTRIC ACID (BETAINE HCL)

Gastric acid, a source of hydrochloric acid, has two major functions. It sterilizes the food and also increases the digestive enzymes if taken with food to improve digestion and help heal leaky gut syndrome. However, if the digestive enzymes are taken on an empty stomach they will have an anti-inflammatory action. It also increases the denaturing proteins—breaking of many of the weak hydrogen bonds within a protein molecule—which prepares the protein for breakdown by gastric and pancreatic enzymes.

Cause

Low levels of hydrochloric acid (hypochlorhydria) in the stomach are caused by widespread use of antacids (which are the third most common OTC medication), prescription drugs that block stomach acid production, the aging process, and also genetic causes. Low stomach acid is also more common in individuals that are vegetarian and in people who fast. In fact, if you have any debilitating chronic condition, it increases your risk of low stomach acid.

Signs and Symptoms

The possible consequences of low stomach acid are significant, including major minerals deficiencies (calcium, magnesium, zinc, iron, chromium, manganese, copper, and molybdenum). Furthermore, B12 deficiency is a possible side effect of low stomach acid. In addition, you may have even more signs and symptoms if you have low stomach acid, such as:

- Acne
- Bloating or belching immediately after meals
- Chronic intestinal infections

- Dilated blood vessels in the cheeks and nose
- Multiple food allergies
- Muscle cramps and spasms

- Rosacea
- Undigested food in your stools
- Upper digestive tract gassiness

Diseases/Conditions Linked to Low Levels

Maintaining low levels of stomach acid can bring about a range of distressing side effects and leave the body exposed to the development of a number of disorders. The following are diseases associated with low stomach acid:

- Acne
- Addison's disease
- Asthma
- Celiac disease
- Chronic candida infections
- Chronic hives
- Chronic parasitic infection
- Dermatitis herpetiformis
- Diabetes mellitus
- Dysbiosis
- Eczema
- Gallbladder disease
- Hepatitis
- Hyper- and hypothyroidism
- Iron deficiency anemia
- Lupus erythematosus
- Myasthenia gravis
- Osteoporosis
- Pernicious anemia
- Psoriasis
- Rheumatoid arthritis
- Rosacea
- Sjogren's syndrome
- Small bowel overgrowth (SIBO)
- Thyrotoxicosis
- Vitiligo

Natural Treatments

Therapies for low stomach acid are contingent on the underlying cause. However, there are some approaches you can try at home to improve stomach acid levels. Below are natural ways to increase hydrochloric acid in the stomach:

- Apple cider vinegar and lemon
- Betaine HCL (do not use if you have a peptic ulcer)
- Bitter herbs
- Chew food thoroughly
- Digestive enzymes
- Enteric-coated peppermint oil
- Garlic
- Ginger
- Glutamine
- Grapefruit seed extract
- Lemons

- Limes
- Multivitamin
- Oregano oil
- Papaya

- Pineapple
- Probiotics
- Vitamin B complex

Work with your healthcare provider to try and avoid use of antacids, PPIs, and H2 receptor antagonists unless you have Barrett's esophagitis. If you have Barrett's esophagitis, then PPIs should be taken for the remainder of your life. If you and your doctor decide to stop your PPI, you may need to wean off of it due to a possible rebound effect if you have been taking it long-term. If you have an H. Pylori infection see your doctor for treatment.

Protocol For HCL Acid Supplementation

You may need to take HCL acid. The following is a protocol for HCL acid supplementation as well as testing to see if you are low in acid. Do not take it if you have an active ulcer or have Barrett's esophagitis or are actively bleeding anywhere.

Begin by taking one tablet or capsule containing 10 grains (600 mg) of HCL at your large next meal. If this does not aggravate your symptoms, at every meal after that of the same size take one more tablet or capsule—one at the next meal, two at the meal after that, then three at the next meal. Continue to increase the dose until you reach seven tablets or when you feel a warmth in your stomach, whichever occurs first. A feeling of warmth in the stomach means that you have taken too many tablets for that meal, and you need to take one less tablet for that meal size. It is a good idea to try the larger dose again at another meal to make sure that it was the HCL that caused the warmth and not something else.

After you have found the largest dose that you can take at your large meals without feeling any warmth, maintain that dose at all of meals of similar size. You will need to take less at smaller meals. When taking a number of tablets or capsules it is best to take them throughout the meal. As your stomach begins to regain the ability to produce the amount of HCL needed to properly digest your food, you will notice the warm feeling again and will have to cut down the dosage. HCL may be used indefinitely in most individuals.

Bile salts. They are very important in helping to digest fats, fat-soluble vitamins, and essential oils as well as carry waste products from the liver. Bile salts are alkaline and help to maintain adequate bowel flora. Low bile salts lead to poor absorption of iron and calcium. The following are signs and symptoms of low bile salts:

- Bloating, gas, abdominal discomfort—especially after fatty meals
- Chronic constipation
- Dull right-sided fullness several hours after eating
- Fat soluble vitamin deficiency
- Heartburn
- Stools that are consistently pale brown, yellowish, or grayish
- Vague and intermittent abdominal pains

When you take bile salts, only take them for two months. If symptoms return, then go back on them for another two months and then discontinue them. Excessive replacement can lead to greenish-tinged diarrhea with an unpleasant odor. Bile salts come from animal sources so you can have allergic reactions to them.

High-fiber diet. A diet high in fiber can promote an increase in bacterial richness in the gut, thereby preventing conditions and diseases, such as obesity and metabolic syndrome. Likewise, adding in fiber in several different forms supports bowel transit time and motility which aids in eliminating toxins.

3. REPOPULATE

To repopulate or re-inoculate is to restore the balance of good bacteria in your gut which is absolutely crucial to your overall health and having optimal immune function. This phase of the program involves using probiotic foods, fiber-rich foods, and commonly a supplement to help beneficial bacteria flourish.

PROBIOTICS

Begin by repopulating the gut with probiotics, which are good bacteria. They improve the intestinal microbial balance. In addition, reintroduction of good GI *microflora* leaves less space for pathogenic organisms to populate. Specifically, research has found strong associations between strains of *Bifidobacteria* and *Lactobacillus* as well as *Saccharomyces boulardii* and improvements in intestinal cell barrier function and intestinal permeability.

If you have a severely compromised immune system, you should not use live probiotics since the organisms may cross the gut lining and be absorbed.

Instead, use the non-live forms of probiotics. Probiotics play a protective role against the colonization of intestinal pathogenic microbes and increase mucosal integrity by stimulating epithelial cells, which are cells that form a barrier between the inside and outside of your body, protecting against viruses. The following are some of the main functions of probiotics for the body.

■ Functions of Probiotics

Probiotics play a role in restoring your digestive system with good bacteria that will neutralize the harmful microbes. They are believed to:

- Activate regulatory T cells that release IL-10
- Act like natural antibiotics
- Downregulation gut inflammation
- Help digest fats
- Help maintain a beneficial intestinal lining which protects against food allergies
- Help to generate cytokines (proteins that regulate immunity)
- Help with detoxification
- Increase the intestinal and systemic immune response
- Interact with the intestinal epithelial cells (IECs) or immune cells associated with the lamina propria (connective tissue that forms part of the mucous membrane), through Toll-like receptors, and induces the production of different cytokines or chemokines
- Maintain the optimal pH of the intestine
- Make B vitamins
- Make short-chain fatty acids
- Modulate intestinal microbiota by maintaining the balance and suppressing the growth of potential pathogenic bacteria in the gut
- Produce digestive enzymes
- Produce lignins (necessary in the formation of cell walls) to protect against cancer
- Protect against parasites
- Reinforce the intestinal barrier by an increase in mucins (major component of mucus), tight junction proteins, goblet (cells that synthesize and secrete mucus), and paneth cells (cells containing proteins that regulate intestinal flora)

■ Probiotic Rich Foods and Drinks

The following foods and liquids serve as probiotics:

- Buttermilk
- Essene bread (Ezekiel bread)
- Fermented sausages
- Fermented vegetables
- Ginger
- Kimchee
- Kombucha
- Miso
- Natto
- Olives
- Raw pickles
- Raw vinegars
- Raw whey
- Sauerkraut
- Sourdough
- Tempeh
- Yogurt/kefir

As previously discussed, commonly probiotics also need to be taken as a supplement. Supplements should be pharmaceutical grade and contain several different strains of *Lactobacillus* sp, *Streptococcus* sp, and *Bifidobacterium* sp. Some also contain *S. boulardii*. The probiotics should contain between 20 billion and 100 billion organisms.

PREBIOTICS

After one month on probiotics, start prebiotics which are agents that support the growth and integrity of the probiotics. In other words, prebiotics are food for good bacteria since they help the growth of beneficial bacteria. They have been reported to improve the expression of tight junction proteins (helps cells form a barrier that stops molecules from getting through), including occludin and zonulin, thereby decreasing intestinal permeability.

Zonulin is the physiological modulator of tight junctions and is involved in the trafficking of macromolecules in and out of the intestine. The detection of zonulin antibodies suggests the dysregulation of tight junctions. The increased translocation of endotoxins and inflammation induce the degradation of occludin and zonulin, which are responsible for preserving the biochemical balance of the GI tract. In other words, these are markers of tight junction damage.

Other biomarkers of intestinal permeability that can be measured are bacterial endotoxin (LPS) IgG, IgA, IgM which are markers of permeability and dysbiosis. In addition, epithelial cell (cells releasing digestive fluids, enzymes, and acid) damage can be measured by examining actomyosin IgA.

■ Functions of Prebiotics

Prebiotics triggers the growth of health microbes in the gut by:

- Causing a significant change of gut microbiota composition, especially an increase of fecal concentrations of *Bifidobacterium*
- Having a positive effect on energy balance
- Helping with satiety regulation
- Improving general well-being and reduces the incidence of allergic symptoms such as atopic eczema
- Improving stool quality (pH, SCFA, frequency, and consistency)
- Improving the expression of tight junction proteins
- Increasing calcium absorption
- Lowering morning cortisol if it is elevated
- Modulating biomarkers and activities of the immune system
- Reducing incidence of tumors and cancers
- Reducing the risk of gastroenteritis and infections

■ Prebiotic Rich Foods

Prebiotic-enriched diets also have been shown to lower inflammatory mediators and decrease oxidative stress as well as increase the production of beneficial short-chain fatty acids such as butyrate. The following are prebiotic rich foods:

- Asparagus
- Burdock root
- Chicory
- Cottage cheese
- Eggplant
- Garlic
- Green tea
- Honey
- Jerusalem artichokes
- Kefir
- Leeks
- Legumes
- Onions
- Peas
- Yogurt

Furthermore, prebiotics improve glucose sensitivity and help to eliminate body fat as well as lower blood pressure and help to eliminate toxins. They also improve liver function and reduce serum cholesterol. Like probiotics, prebiotics are available commercially in the form of fructo-oligosaccharides (FOS), guar, lactulose, and inulin. Prebiotics are also available in many foods that contain inulin, such as garlic, onions, legumes, chicory, soybeans, asparagus, garlic, and leeks.

You may need to take probiotics and prebiotics for the remainder of your life. The best way to permanently change the gut microbiota in your body is to eat a healthy diet. If you have had a major GI problem, such as surgery to the intestine, then you may want to consider microbiota transplantation if symptoms continue and lab work remains abnormal.

4. REPAIR

The gut lining can be severely damaged during times when the body is inflamed, under stress, and exposed to allergens long-term. This increases the intestinal permeability of the gut which allows antigenic macromolecules to cross the gut epithelium (gut tissue) leading to chronic systemic inflammation, which then decreases the gut bacteria leading to leaky gut syndrome. Repair of the GI tract lining is needed to ensure proper absorption of nutrients as well as medications.

THERAPIES

Repair of the GI lining requires several therapies. Begin by eating a diet rich in amino acids, vitamins, and minerals. The following therapies have also been shown to be beneficial.

- **Anti-inflammatory agents** such as fish oil, which can reverse intestinal dysbiosis, and curcumin, which improves barrier function.

- **Chamomile** (*Matricaria chamomilla*) has anti-inflammatory action that is due to azulene and bisaboline, which are two chemicals in chamomile. Its name means "mother of the gut." In Germany it is an OTC licensed drug for treatment of GI spasms and inflammatory diseases of the GI tract.

- **Chinese skullcap** (*Scutellaria baicalensis*) contains baicalin and wogonin, which have anti-inflammatory action by blocking the arachidonic acid cascade and it helps heal the gastric mucosa.

- **Citrus flavanones** can modulate the microbiota composition, as indicated in recent evidence, and activity by inhibiting pathogenic bacteria and selectively stimulating the growth of good bacteria. Citrus flavanones, with hesperidin and naringin as the most abundant representatives, also have various beneficial effects, including anti-oxidative and anti-inflammatory activities. In addition, the consumption of citrus flavanones has been associated with a lower risk of degenerative diseases, such as cardiovascular diseases and cancers.

- **Demulcents** are herbs or foods that have a protective effect on the mucous membranes of the body. They contain a large amount of mucilaginous materials that have a direct effect on the lining of the intestines to sooth them. Likewise, demulcents also reduce the sensitivity of the digestive system to gastric acids, relax spasms, decrease leaky gut, inflammation, and ulceration. The following are examples of demulcents:

  - Cabbage juice
  - Fenugreek (*Trigonella foenum-graecum*)
  - Marshmallow (*Althea officinalis*)
  - Okra (*Hibiscus esculentus*)
  - Slippery elm bark (*Ulmus fulva*)

- **Ginkgo biloba** has been shown to protect the integrity of the mucosal lining of the intestines by reducing oxidative damage.

- **Goldenseal** (*Hydrastis canadensis*) stimulates the immune response and destroys germs since it contains berberine. It also has astringent effects that aid in digestive problems and is used to treat peptic ulcers and colitis. Goldenseal, in addition, promotes the production and secretion of digestive juices and helps to reestablish healthy gut mucosa. Barberry or Oregon grape root, which are berberine-rich substitutes, can also be used.

- **Glutamine** is an amino acid that stimulates intestinal mucosal growth and protects the gut from mucosal atrophy. It also plays an important role in acid-base balance and has an immunomodulating effect by increasing IL-6 levels and lymphocyte function. However, glutamine is a precursor to glutamate or glutamic acid. Glutamate is one of two excitatory neurotransmitters in the brain that can cause anxiety. Consequently, work with your healthcare provider before taking glutamine. Levels of your amino acids can be measured by blood or urine and then you and your doctor can make an informed decision on the use of glutamine for GI health.

- **Licorice root** (*Glycyrrhiza giabra*), which contains flavonoids called saponin glycosides, have a protective effect on the gut. It has also been shown to decrease GI bleeding secondary to NSAIDs.

- **Meadowsweet** (*Filipendula ulmaria*), contains glycosides, tannins, mucilage, and flavonoids, which acts as an anti-inflammatory. In addition, it aids in strengthening the bonds of the connective tissue between cells, which helps protect the intestinal barrier. It is also a free radical scavenger.

- **Mucosal secretion,** such as phosphatidylcholine, plantain, and polysaccharides, protects the respiratory system with lubrication and plays an important role in the allergic inflammatory response.

- **Nutrients** that are antioxidants, such as carotenoids, and vitamins A, C, D, E, selenium, and zinc along with n-acetyl cysteine (NAC), decrease oxidative stress, which is one of the main causes of intestinal damage.

- **Phosphatidylcholine** (PC) is a ubiquitous membrane phospholipid that is essential for cellular differentiation, proliferation, and regeneration and is necessary for the transport of molecules through membranes. It has been shown to improve intestinal barrier function.

  DOSE: 1,000 mg a day. If you have elevated TMAO levels do not take PC.

- **Quercetin** is a bioflavonoid that is found in onions and blue-green algae. It is an antioxidant and an anti-inflammatory, and it works by decreasing mast cell (acts as an anticoagulant) and basophil (type of white blood cell) production.

- **Whey, immunoglobulins, lactoferrin, and lactoperoxidase** support gut-associated lymphoid tissue (GALT) function.

ENERGY BALANCE

The ability to repair is also affected by energy balance. Anything that affects ATPase activity (necessary for cell metabolism and exporting toxins) can also affect absorption. The ATPase activity and absorption of nutrients can be impacted by a magnesium deficiency, insulin resistance, hypothyroidism (low thyroid function), catecholamine production (hormones and neurotransmitters by the adrenal glands and other organs), and adrenal insufficiency by altering glucocorticoid (steroid) metabolism.

5. REBALANCE

Rebalance, the 5th R in the program, is where your way of life plays a crucial role. It is necessary to address the external stressors in your life that may increase your sympathetic drive in the nervous system and reduce the parasympathetic drive. The sympathetic section generally functions in actions requiring quick responses, fight or flight. The parasympathetic section functions with actions that do not require immediate reaction, associated with relaxation, digestion, and regeneration.

With practices like yoga, meditation, deep breathing, good sleep and other mindfulness-based practices, you can help restore hormone balance that will protect your gut and subsequently, your entire body. It would be pointless to go through the first 4 R's of the gut restoration program to only go back to old eating habits, lack of exercise, stress, and other things that contributed to the GI dysfunction. The 5th R is just as important as the others for optimal GI health.

THE GI TRACT AND THE IMMUNE SYSTEM

The mucosal immune system of the GI tract both controls the GI microbiome and depends on it. The mucosal immune responses take place at mucosal membranes of the intestines, the urogenital tract, and the respiratory system. The permanent challenge of bacterial antigens to the mucosal immune system is required for its normal development and function. Therefore, it is not surprising that the GI immune system contains cells capable of recognizing bacterial antigens by specific receptors. These include:

- Dendritic cells (via TLRs)

- Innate immune cells, such as macrophages and mast cells (via TLRs and other PRRs)

- Lymphocytes (via TCRs and antibodies)

- Pattern recognition receptors (PRRs) of the innate immune system

- Surface-bound antibodies of the adaptive immune system

- T cell receptors (TCRs) and B cell-derived

- Toll-like receptors (TLRs)

All of these are additionally involved in the communication between the GI microbiome and the GI immune system so that any danger from pathogens can be recognized. Likewise, they help maintain friendly gut flora. These immune markers were discussed in Part 1 of this book.

Moreover, to achieve the defense of the host against luminal bacteria and other potentially harmful substances, the GI immune system is equipped with tools, such as: plasma cell-dependent immunoglobulin A (IgA) defense system, goblet cell-derived mucus production, synthesis of antimicrobial peptides, such as defensins (proteins) by Paneth cells in the small intestine epithelium (membranous tissue).

When exposed to bacteria or bacterial antigens, Paneth cells secrete compounds into the lumen of the intestinal gland, thereby contributing to maintenance of the gastrointestinal barrier. All of these play a part in controlling the

GI microbiome and protecting the host against invasion of luminal bacteria through the gut wall. In healthy people, these mechanisms also prevent direct contact between natural bacteria and the GI epithelium.

Furthermore, the GI immune system allows regulation of inflammatory responses to harmless antigens, such as food antigens or bacterial antigens derived from commensals (organisms that derive food or other benefits from another organism without hurting or helping it), by mechanisms that together result in mucosal tolerance.

If there is loss of the bacterial challenge and immune tolerance just described, it results in intense hypersensitivity reactions, which lead to chronic inflammatory states, such as allergies, autoimmune diseases, and inflammatory bowel disease. Therefore, the GI immune system contributes to both the defense against, and the acceptance of, bacteria and it wards off bacteria, but still needs them. All these functions exemplify the complex balance of interactions between the GI microbiome and the GI immune system.

CONCLUSION

This chapter has explored the importance of normal GI microbiota, which is of rich diversity, as well as the significance of an intact GI barrier. Both are needed to maintain optimal gut health. Therefore, the intestinal microbiota has many functions that are important for your health. During normal intestinal homeostasis, the balance between inhibiting invading pathogens and tolerance to commensal microbes is tightly regulated. However, a disturbed barrier function and/or reduced tolerance may facilitate intestinal inflammation. As part of the inflammatory response, reactive oxygen species and reactive nitrogen species are produced, resulting in enhanced exposure to oxidative stress.

In review, a healthy gut flora supports optimal digestion of food, hormone balance, and immune function. It helps to maintain optimal levels of vitamins and minerals, balances neurotransmitter levels, and reduces inflammation. The mechanisms of ensuring gut health are complex and comprise a healthy lifestyle, a balanced diet, normal GI perfusion, and normal GI microbiota along with the remainder of the items discussed in this chapter.

The key to understanding gut health is an awareness that the GI barrier consists of multiple epithelial functions as well as the mucosal immune system. The GI barrier not only protects you against potential dangers from the GI lumen, but also allows food and liquid uptake, beneficial cross-talk to the good bacteria, and immune tolerance against harmless antigens. An intact GI barrier maintains gut health. Whereas disturbance of GI barrier (leaky gut syndrome) is increasingly recognized as an early but important step in the pathogenesis of various illnesses both directly related to the GI tract and also other parts of the body as well. The management of gut flora to enrich its protective and beneficial role represents a promising field of new therapeutic strategies focused on prevention and treatment of many disease processes along with enhancement of the immune system.

8

Inflammation

Its Effect on
the Immune System

nflammation is a signal-mediated response to cellular insult by infectious agents, smoking, toxins, physical stresses, and even elevated cholesterol. As a crucial part of the immune system's response to injury and infection, inflammation signals the immune system to heal and repair damaged tissue. Consequently, healthy immune systems use inflammation to fix an unbalanced body. A small amount of inflammation heals however too much inflammation is linked to many major diseases. Therefore, inflammation has a major impact on the immune system. When you run a temperature after catching a cold or have bronchitis, when you have a cough or have other symptoms, they are related to the body's inflammatory process setting up a healing response. It also assists in building long-term adaptive immunity towards some microbes.

Inflammation is the key to every major disease that occurs in the body after the age of 45 and of many other diseases that occur in younger individuals. Most medical treatments are centered on resolving symptoms and not looking at the cause or etiology of the signs, symptoms, and illness itself. This chapter will focus on the balancing of the inflammatory response.

The body sets up an inflammatory response to try and accomplish three goals:

1. To defend itself against an infection, such as a virus, bacteria, parasite, or fungus

2. To set up a detoxification mechanism

3. To heal itself

ACUTE/CHRONIC INFLAMMATION

There are two types of inflammation: acute and chronic. Acute inflammation is the body immediately trying to repair itself from injury or infection. It is the initial response to damaging stimuli, achieved by an increased mobility of plasma and leukocytes from the blood into the impaired tissue. You may experience swelling, pain, redness, or loss of function. Chronic inflammation is an ongoing response of the immune system to a problem. Long-term inflammation may last for many years and even a lifetime. It can take place even when there is no injury, and it does not always come to an end when you recover from the illness or injury. While acute inflammation is important to the immune response, chronic inappropriate inflammation can cause tissue destruction. This increases the risk of developing an autoimmune disease (a condition where your immune system mistakenly attacks your body), a neuro-degenerative disorder, or cardiovascular disease.

To more be specific, inflammation is a biological response of the immune system that can be triggered by a variety of factors, including pathogens, damaged cells, and toxic compounds. These factors may induce acute and/or chronic inflammatory responses in the heart, pancreas, liver, kidney, lung, brain, intestinal tract, reproductive system, as well as other organs and tissues potentially leading to damage or disease. Both infectious and non-infectious vehicles as well as cell damage activate inflammatory cells and trigger inflammatory signaling pathways. The most common pathways are the NF-kB, MAPK, and JAK-STAT pathways discussed in the first section of this book.

WHAT CAUSES INFLAMMATION IN THE BODY?

Before the body sets up an inflammatory response, the immune system has to recognize a threat to the body from one or more of the following categories that are discussed at length in Dr. Nancy Appleton's book entitled: *Stopping Inflammation: Relieving the Cause of Degenerative Diseases.*

- Microbial infections: viruses, bacteria, parasites, fungi infections can set up an inflammatory response by secreting various white blood cells

- Surgery: of any type including oral surgery

- Physical agents: tissue damage can occur due to trauma, ultraviolet or other form of radiation, burns, or frostbite

- Vaccinations: all cause an inflammatory response

- Chemicals: from household cleaners, products at work, pesticides, products during traveling

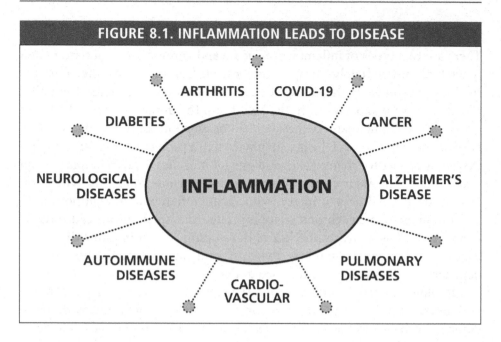

FIGURE 8.1. INFLAMMATION LEADS TO DISEASE

- Disease processes: most diseases after the age of 45 and many diseases when you are younger

- Smoking and other tobacco use: sets up an inflammatory response (*see* chapter 10)

- AGEs: advances glycation end products are a source of inflammation from the diet and eating processed foods

- Free radical production: cause oxidative stress which creates inflammation

- Obesity: the more overweight you are the more inflamed you are

- Chronic fatigue: puts stress on the body which produces inflammation

- Allergies: to foods, spices, and environmental vehicles, such as trees, animal dander, pollen

In addition, other causes of inflammation have also been discussed in the medical literature.

- Dairy products
- Disrupted circadian rhythms (abnormal sleeping pattern, see chapter on sleep)
- Histamine intolerance syndrome

- Imbalanced diet
- Medications
- Mitochondrial damage
- Physical inactivity

WHAT HAPPENS TO THE BODY
IN AN INFLAMMATORY REACTION

The primary goal of the inflammatory response is to detect and eliminate factors that interfere with homeostasis. A typical inflammatory response consists of four components: inflammatory inducers; the detecting sensors; downstream mediators; and the target tissues that are affected.

The type and the degree of inflammatory response activated is dependent on the nature of the inflammatory trigger (bacterial, viral, or parasitic) and its persistence. The body produces substances to try and decrease the inflammation and attempt to heal itself.

A healthy person produces circulating immune complexes. They are made up of the foreign invader or antigen and white blood cells called antibodies. The following are some of the inflammatory mediators produced by the body.

- Chemokines
- Cytokines
- Eosinophils
- Free radical production
- Insulin

- Interleukins
- Leukotrienes
- Mast cells
- Prostaglandins
- Serotonin

Physical Changes

The classic signs of inflammation are heat, redness, swelling, pain, and loss of function. These are manifestations of the physiologic changes that occur during the inflammatory process. The three major components of this process are (1) changes in the caliber of blood vessels and the rate of blood flow through them (hemodynamic changes); (2) increased capillary permeability; and (3) leukocytic exudation which is fluid that filters from the circulatory system into areas of inflammation.

To explain this process further, hemodynamic changes begin soon after injury and progress at varying rates, according to the extent of injury. They start with dilation of the arterioles and the opening of new capillaries and venular beds—small branches of a vein—in the area. This causes an accelerated flow of blood, accounting for the signs of heat and redness. Next follows increased permeability of the microcirculation, which permits leakage of protein-rich fluid out of small blood vessels and into the extravascular fluid compartment, accounting for the inflammatory edema. Leukocytic release occurs in the following sequence:

1. First, the leukocytes move to the endothelial lining of the small blood vessels and line the endothelium in a tightly packed formation.

2. Subsequently, these leukocytes move through the endothelial spaces and escape outside the blood vessels where they are free to move and, by chemotaxis, are drawn to the area of injury.

3. Accumulations of neutrophils and macrophages at the area of inflammation then act to neutralize foreign particles by a process called phagocytosis.

Chemical Mediators

Chemical mediators of the inflammatory process include a variety of substances originating in the plasma and the cells of uninjured tissue, and possibly from the damaged tissue. These kinds of mediators are the following:

- Lymphocyte factors

- Neutrophil products

- Plasma endopeptidases that comprise three systems that are interrelated

- Kinin system that makes bradykinin (a peptide causing blood cells to dilate or enlarge)

- Clotting system that increases vascular permeability and chemotactic activity for the leukocytes

- Complement system that produces proteins that interact with antigen-antibody complexes and mediate immunologic injury and inflammation

- Prostaglandins, which can produce several features of the inflammatory process

- Vasoactive amines, such as histamine and serotonin

- Other factors, such as slow-reacting substance of anaphylaxis and endogenous pyrogens

A hormonal response also occurs where hormones such as cortisol are produced, which have an anti-inflammatory effect. Some other hormones have a pro-inflammatory effect. Thus, the endocrine system has a regulatory effect on the process of inflammation so that it can be balanced and beneficial in the body's attempts to recover from injury or infection.

ALLERGIES AND INFLAMMATION

There is a strong link between allergies and inflammation. The symptoms of allergies that arise from inflammation are caused by uncontrolled chemicals that are released from cells in an erroneous attempt to protect the body, as well as foods, exposure to chemicals, and even stress.

Allergic inflammation is complex, involving many cells and mediators. Allergic inflammation is mediated by Th2 and Th9 lymphocytes and their products, IgE and mast cells, eosinophils, basophils, and epithelial cells. Innate immunity, involving epithelial cells producing IL-25, IL-33 and TSLP (a protein) as well as NKT (natural killer T) cells producing Th2 cytokines may contribute to this inflammation.

Food Allergies

There are three responses that you can have to food, which include food allergy, food sensitivity, and food intolerance.

1. Food Allergy

Food allergy is an immunologic hypersensitivity response which is an IgE antibody reaction. It is an immediate response (usually occurs within seconds or minutes) to an antigen that has entered the body. IgE responses are associated with mast cell production and histamine release. Symptoms include the following:

- Anaphylactic shock (in severe cases)
- Anxiety
- Hives
- Inflammation
- Itching
- Rash
- Reddened earlobes, eyes, or checks
- Shortness of breath
- Swelling
- Throat tightening

2. Food Sensitivity

Food sensitivity is an immunologic delayed reaction to food which is an IgG reaction. Symptoms of IgG reactions usually occur in 24 to 72 hours after eating the food, are more subtle, and can last much longer than a traditional IgE response. IgG antibodies lead to inflammatory processes and are not associated with the release of histamine, so you will not get the immediate hypersensitivity reaction that you get with an actual food allergy.

- Abdominal pain
- Anal itching

- Anemia
- Asthma
- Backache
- Canker sores
- Chest pain
- Cracks on corners of the mouth
- Dark circles under the eyes
- Diarrhea
- Dizziness
- Eczema
- Fatigue
- Fluid retention
- Food cravings
- Frequent urination
- Gas
- Headaches: both tension and non-tension

- Heart palpitations
- Heartburn
- Hoarseness
- Itchy, watery eyes
- Itchy skin
- Low blood pressure
- Muscle aches
- Nasal congestion
- Nausea
- Persistent cough
- Tinnitus (ringing in the ears)
- Sinusitis
- Sniffing and sneezing
- Stomach cramps
- Tremors
- Wrinkles under the eyes

3. Food Intolerance

Food intolerance is a non-immunological response. It is estimated that up to 20 percent of people in the United States have food intolerances. Symptoms of food intolerance include the following:

- Bloating
- Diarrhea
- Gas
- Malaise

- Migraine headaches
- Runny nose
- Stomach pain

Environmental Allergies

Environmental allergies are a response to triggers you come in contact with that exist in your surroundings, indoor or outdoor. The most common causes of *indoor allergies* are cigarette smoke, cleaning products, cosmetics, dust mites, mold, hairsprays, laundry detergents, perfume, pet hair or dander, and soaps.

The most common *outdoor allergens* are air pollutants, chlorine, diesel exhaust, hay fever, insect bites and stings, mold, poison ivy, oak, or sumac. The following signs and symptoms are related to environmental allergies.

- Cough
- Decreased hand-eye coordination
- Fatigue
- Headache
- Inability to concentrate and make decisions
- Irritability
- Itchy eyes, mouth or skin

- Puffy, swollen eyelids
- Runny nose
- Shortness of breath
- Sleep disorders
- Sneezing
- Stuffy nose due to congestion or nasal blockage
- Wheezing

Therapies for both food and environment allergies range from medications to over-the-counter drugs, to nutrients, such as quercetin, Boswellia, curcumin, perilla, and stinging nettle. Of course, avoidance of the food you are allergic to, or have a sensitivity to, is the place to begin if you have food allergies, along with avoiding the indoor or outdoor allergens if you suffer from environmental allergies.

LEAKY GUT SYNDROME AND INFLAMMATION

Leaky gut syndrome results from continuous damage to the gastrointestinal tract (GI) from inflammatory processes due to infection, to antibiotic use, to food allergies. If your GI tract is not healthy, commonly there is inflammation being displayed as part of this reaction. When you suffer from a leaky gut, bacteria and toxins enter the blood stream and can cause inflammation and may bring about a reaction from the immune system. *See* chapter 7 on GI health for a more extensive discussion.

ADVANCED GLYCATION END PRODUCTS (AGEs)

There are also other forms of inflammation that are important to further examine. Advanced glycation end products (AGEs), found in protein-rich and sugar-rich foods, can attack any part of the body and mimic a low-grade infection. Advanced glycation end products are proteins or lipids that become glycated as a result of exposure to sugars. They are a biomarker implicated in aging and the development, or worsening, of many diseases.

Conditions Caused By AGEs

AGEs accumulate naturally as you age and high levels have been connected to the development of many diseases. The following are such conditions that can be caused by AGEs.

- Atherosclerosis
- Cancer growth
- Cataracts
- Decreased ability of blood vessels to dilate
- Decreased ability of fats to be cleared from the body
- Diabetes
- Hypertension
- Increased blood clotting

- Increased oxidative stress
- Inflammation
- Joint stiffness
- Macular degeneration
- Memory loss including Alzheimer's disease and other forms of dementia
- Rheumatoid arthritis
- Uremia and other forms of kidney damage

Once AGE products are formed, they are not reversible. As glycation begins, free radicals form in glycated products at five times the rate of non-glycated proteins. Free radicals produce inflammation and oxidative stress.

FREE RADICALS

Immune cells produce free radicals while fighting off antigens that are invading the body. A free radical is a molecule that contains an unpaired electron which is in search of another electron to stabilize the molecule. Oxygen-derived free radicals are important in both natural and acquired immunity. Neutrophil and macrophage phagocytosis stimulates various cellular processes including the "respiratory burst," whereby increased cellular oxygen uptake results in the production of potent oxidant bactericidal agents. In addition, nitric oxide, a gaseous radical produced by macrophages, reacts with superoxide to form peroxynitrite, which is also a potent bactericidal (kills bacteria) agent.

On the other hand, oxidative stress may be detrimental in acquired immunity by activation of nuclear factor kappa B, which governs gene expression involving, for example, various cytokines, chemokines, and cell adhesion molecules. Inflammation that is unregulated creates free radical production.

SOURCES OF FREE RADICAL PRODUCTION

Although free radicals are produced naturally in the body, factors contributed to your environment and lifestyle influence their production. The following are sources of free radical production.

General factors

- Aging process
- Chronic stress (Who is not stressed in today's world?)
- Normal metabolism of the body

Dietary factors

- Additives
- Alcohol in excessive amounts (more than one drink a day for a female and more than two drinks a day for a male)
- Caffeine
- Fried foods
- Herbicides and pesticides
- Hydrogenated vegetable oils
- Sugar, sugar, and sugar!

Chemical factors

- Air pollutants
- Chemical pollutants
- Cosmic radiation
- Electromagnetic fields (Besides sugar, electromagnetic fields may be the largest producer of free radicals.)
- Flying in an airplane
- Medical and dental x-rays
- Radiation

The good news is that taking antioxidants and eating foods that function as antioxidants can reverse several age-associated immune deficiencies. This results in increased levels of interleukin-2, elevated numbers of total lymphocytes and T cell subsets, enhanced mitogen responsiveness, increased killer cell activity, augmented antibody response to antigen stimulation, decreased lipid peroxidation, and decreased prostaglandin synthesis. As previously discussed, damaging free radicals can also cause the production of oxidation and inflammation.

DISEASES RELATED TO INFLAMMATION

Inflammation plays a central role in healing, but chronic inflammation raises the risk of certain diseases. In fact, most diseases that occur after the age of 45 are inflammatory in nature. Long-term disease processes that are attributed in the medical literature to inflammation may include the following:

- Allergy
- Alzheimer's disease and other forms of cognitive decline
- Asthma
- Diabetes
- Cancer
- Candida infections
- Canker sores and mouth ulcers
- Cardiovascular disease
- COVID-19
- Depression
- Epilepsy
- Food addictions and eating disorders
- Headaches
- Heartburn
- Hypertension
- Hypoglycemia
- Inflammatory bowel disease
- Kidney disease
- Lyme disease
- Obesity
- Parkinson's disease
- Periodontal disease
- Respiratory diseases
- Rheumatoid arthritis

An entire book could be written, and has been written, concerning disease and inflammation. I would like to discuss four examples—obesity, cardiovascular disease, tumor development, severe acute respiratory syndromes—from the above list to showcase how inflammation plays a role in these disease processes.

Obesity

The visceral fat contains a rich blood and nerve supply as well as pro-inflammatory molecules, such as interleukin 6 (IL-6), tumor necrosis factor alpha (TNF alpha), leptin, and resistin, the adipocytokines, and acute phase proteins (APP). These are activated from adipocytes—cells that primarily compose adipose tissue that specializes in storing energy as fat—and/or macrophages by sympathetic signaling. The inflammation is linked to fat accumulation. Over the last decade, an abundance of evidence has emerged demonstrating a close link between metabolism and immunity. It is now clear that obesity is associated with a state of chronic low-level inflammation and subsequent compromised immunity.

Cardiovascular Disease (CVD)

Cardiovascular disease (CVD) is the leading cause of mortality worldwide, accounting for 16.7 million deaths each year. The underlying cause of the majority of CVD is atherosclerosis. In the past, atherosclerosis was considered to be the result of passive lipid accumulation in the vessel wall. Current research reveals that cardiovascular disease is a more complex picture than previously believed.

Atherosclerosis is considered a chronic inflammatory disease that results in the formation of plaques in large and mid-sized arteries. Both cells of the innate and the adaptive immune system play a crucial role in its development. By transforming immune cells into pro- and anti-inflammatory chemokine- and cytokine-producing units, and by guiding the interactions between the different immune cells, the immune system significantly influences the propensity of plaque to rupture and cause clinical symptoms, such as a heart attack or stroke.

Tumor Development

Inflammatory responses play decisive roles at different stages of tumor development, including initiation, promotion, malignant conversion, invasion, and metastasis. Inflammation also affects immune surveillance and responses to therapy. Immune cells that infiltrate tumors engage in an extensive and dynamic crosstalk with cancer cells.

Epigenetic disorders—caused by modifications of gene expression in organisms—such as point mutations in cellular tumor suppressor genes, DNA methylation, and post-translational modifications are needed to transform normal cells into cancer cells. These events result in alterations in crucial pathways that when altered trigger an inflammatory response which can lead the development of cancer.

Many inflammatory signaling pathways are activated in several types of cancer, linking chronic inflammation to the tumorigenesis process. Immune cells that infiltrate tumors engage in an extensive crosstalk with cancer cells. A range of inflammation mediators, including cytokines, chemokines, free radicals, prostaglandins, growth and transcription factors, microRNAs, and enzymes as, cyclooxygenase and matrix metalloproteinase, collectively act to create a favorable microenvironment for the development of tumors.

Severe Acute Respiratory Syndromes (SARS-CoV-2)

Severe acute respiratory syndrome coronavirus 2 (SARS-CoV-2) is the causative agent of the coronavirus disease 2019 (COVID-19) pandemic. The host immune response, including innate and adaptive immunity against SARS-Cov-2, appears crucial to control and resolve the viral infection. However, the severity and outcome of the COVID-19 may be associated with the excessive production of pro-inflammatory cytokines otherwise known as "cytokine storm," which can lead to acute respiratory distress syndrome.

Inflammation is a physiological response to infections and tissue injury; it initiates pathogen killing as well as tissue repair processes and helps to restore homeostasis at infected or damaged sites. Acute inflammatory reactions are usually self-limiting and therefore resolve rapidly. Regulating inflammatory responses are essential to staying healthy and maintain balance in the body. Conversely, inflammatory responses that fail to regulate themselves can become chronic and contribute to the perpetuation and progression of disease.

Characteristics typical of chronic inflammatory responses include: loss of barrier function, responsiveness to a normally benign stimulus, infiltration of inflammatory cells into compartments where they are not normally found in large numbers, and overproduction of oxidants, cytokines, chemokines, eicosanoids—signaling molecules—and matrix metalloproteinases—protease enzyme whose catalytic mechanism involves metal. The levels of these mediators amplify the inflammatory response and are destructive. They also contribute to the clinical symptoms.

COMMON TESTS FOR INFLAMMATION

There are now several blood tests that your healthcare provider can order that will help determine if your body is inflamed. Such tests should be performed regularly as a preventative action and to monitor your inflammatory standing.

CRP blood test. C-reactive protein levels rise acutely in response to inflammation following IL-6 secretion by macrophages and T cells. Its physiological role is to bind to the surface of dead or dying cells (and some types of bacteria) in order to activate the complement system.

Interleukin-6 blood test. Interleukin-6 (IL-6) is an interleukin that acts as both a pro-inflammatory cytokine and an anti-inflammatory myokine mediated through its inhibitory effects on TNF-alpha and IL-1. This blood test helps to evaluate conditions, such as lupus, rheumatoid arthritis or even infection, which is linked to inflammation.

TNF-alpha blood test. TNF-alpha is a cell signaling protein (cytokine) involved in systemic inflammation and is one of the cytokines that makes up the acute phase reaction. It is produced chiefly by activated macrophages, although it can be produced by many other cell types, such as T helper cells, natural killer cells, neutrophils, mast cells, eosinophils, and neurons.

Cytokine profile test. Cytokines include chemokines, interferons, interleukins, lymphokines, and tumor necrosis factors. Cytokines are produced by a broad range of cells, including immune cells like macrophages, B lymphocytes, T lymphocytes and mast cells, as well as endothelial cells, fibroblasts, and various stromal cells—cells found in bone marrow. They act through cell surface receptors and they modulate the balance between humoral and cell-based immune responses. Cytokines are involved in host immune responses to infection, inflammation, trauma, sepsis, cancer, and reproduction.

Interleukin-2 blood test. Interleukin-2 (IL-2) is an interleukin, a type of cytokine signaling molecule in the immune system. It regulates the activities of white blood cells (leukocytes and lymphocytes) that are responsible for immunity and it is part of the body's response to microbial infection. The major sources of IL-2 are activated CD4+ T cells and activated CD8+ T cells.

Leukotriene test. Leukotrienes are a family of eicosanoid inflammatory mediators produced in leukocytes by the oxidation of arachidonic acid (AA) and the essential fatty acid eicosapentaenoic acid (EPA). Leukotrienes regulate immune responses and their production is usually accompanied by the manufacturing of histamine and prostaglandins, which also act as inflammatory mediators. Depending on what country you live in, different tests are available to measure leukotrienes in the body.

Erythrocyte sedimentation rate (sed rate). Sed rate is a common blood study that is a non-specific measure of inflammation.

Fibrinogen blood test. Fibrinogen is an acute-phase protein produced by the liver. Its blood levels rise in response to systemic inflammation, tissue injury, and certain other metabolic events such as cancer. High levels are related to thrombosis (clotting) and vascular injury.

Histamine blood test. Histamine is produced by basophils and by mast cells and is involved in local immune responses, as well as regulation of physiological function in the gut. In addition, histamine acts as a neurotransmitter for the brain, spinal cord, and uterus. Furthermore, histamine is involved in the inflammatory response and has a central role as a mediator of itching. It also increases the permeability of the capillaries to white blood cells and some proteins, which allows them to activate against pathogens in infected tissues. Histamine levels can also be measured in the urine and in the stool.

Eosinophils blood test. Eosinophils are a type of white blood cell and they play two roles in your immune system. They destroy foreign substances and regulate inflammation. Levels commonly elevate due to allergic reactions and parasitic and fungal infections. Levels may also rise in autoimmune disorders, skin diseases, and cancer.

GlycA test. GlycA is newer blood marker that tracks systemic inflammation and subclinical vascular inflammation.

TREATMENTS

Research is beginning to show evidence that inflammation could be a factor in a wide variety of diseases and illnesses. Fortunately, there are now conventional, personalized therapies—diet and herbal and nutritional—remedies that present scientific promise.

Conventional Medicine Therapies

Conventional therapies are centered on non-steroidal anti-inflammatory drugs (NSAIDs) that are both prescriptions and non-prescriptions, steroids, and second tier medications that are immune-suppressants and hydroxychloroquine.

Prescription and Non-prescription

- Hydroxychloroquine
- NSAIDs
- Steroids

Immunosuppressants. The following are examples of this class of drugs:

- 6-mercaptopurine
- Azathioprine
- Cyclosporine
- Methotrexate
- Tacrolimus

Personalized Medicine Therapies

You don't have to rely solely on prescription and non-prescription drugs to decrease inflammation. Improving your lifestyle can balance inflammation in the body as well. It's possible to enhance your immunity the healthy way, by improving your diet and taking certain vitamins and herbal preparation.

Diet. Proper nutrition and a balanced diet can be fundamental in preventing ill-ness, from a common cold to cancer. Dietary patterns high in refined starches, sugar, and saturated and trans-fatty acids and poor in natural antioxidants and fiber from fruits, vegetables, and whole grains, as well as poor in omega-3-fatty acids may cause an activation of the innate immune system. Most likely this is due to an excessive production of proinflammatory cytokines associated with a reduced production of anti-inflammatory cytokines. Higher intake of fruit and vegetables lead to both a reduction in pro-inflammatory mediators and an enhanced immune cell profile. Avoiding the use of sugar or the intake of sugary foods and beverages can help to decrease inflammation. *See* chapter 12 on sugar.

Herbal Therapies and Nutrients. Various dietary components including long chain Omega-3 fatty acids, antioxidant vitamins, plant flavonoids, prebiotics and probiotics have the potential to modulate your predisposition to chronic inflammatory conditions. These components act through a variety of mech-anisms including decreasing inflammatory mediator production through effects on cell signaling and gene expression (omega-3 fatty acids, vitamin E, plant flavonoids). In addition, it reduces the production of damaging oxidants (vitamin E and other antioxidants), and it promotes gut barrier function and anti-inflammatory responses (prebiotics and probiotics). Common anti-in-flammatory herbal plants are discussed in Part 3 of this book.

OMEGA-3 FATTY ACIDS

Nutritionally omega-3-fatty acids are the keystone of anti-inflammatory ther-apy. Omega-3-fatty acids are used in the formation of cell membranes, assist in circulation and oxygen uptake, reduce inflammation, and do so much more. There are eleven different types of omega-3-fatty acids. The most important of them are alpha-linolenic acid (ALA), docosahexaenoic acid (DHA) and eicosapentaenoic acid (EPA). The body is able to convert ALA into EPA and DHA, although this conversion process is not efficient and can produce only small amounts of EPA and DHA. ALA cannot be produced by the body, but fortunately, most people in industrialized countries get adequate amounts of this fatty acid from the foods they eat.

Functions of Omega-3-Fatty Acids in Your Body

Omega-3 fatty acids perform various important tasks in your body and pro-vide several health benefits, such as:

- Crucial for many brain functions

- Decreases inflammation
- Decreases rate of arrhythmias (irregular heartbeat)
- Diminishes build-up of plaque in arteries
- Enhances insulin function
- Helps convert nutrients from food into usable forms of energy
- Improves immune function in infants
- Involved in cell-to-cell communication
- Is an important component of brain structure and function
- Is important for mitochondrial function (which produces energy for the cells)
- Lowers triglycerides
- Makes blood less "sticky" and less likely to form dangerous clots
- May decrease homocysteine levels, decreasing the risk for heart disease
- May help treat depression
- May protect against ischemic heart disease (decreased blood flow to the heart)
- May protect the brain from stroke
- Necessary for the normal development and function of the adrenal glands, brain, eyes, inner ear, and reproductive tract
- Needed to make certain prostaglandins—hormones that affect inflammation, decrease menstrual cramps, and increase immune function
- Provides structural support for the membranes of the cell
- Raises HDL (good) cholesterol
- Reduces premenstrual syndrome (PMS) symptoms
- Used to manufacture red blood cells

■ Signs and Symptoms of Omega-3-Fatty Acid Deficiency

Omega-3 fatty acid is one type of fat you do not want to cut back on. Your cells need omega-3- fatty acids and a deficiency signifies that your body is not obtaining enough omega-3 fats. This may put you in danger of negative health effects. The following are potential signs and symptoms of omega-3-fatty acid deficiency.

- Allergies
- Arthritis
- Asthma
- Behavioral changes
- Brittle nails
- Bumps on the upper arm
- Cognitive decline
- Craving fatty foods
- Dandruff
- Depression
- Dry skin
- Excessive urination
- Growth retardation
- Hair loss
- Impaired immune response
- Impaired motor coordination
- Inflammation
- Learning disorders
- Mood swings
- Thirst
- Tingling feeling in arms or legs

■ Causes of Omega-3-Fatty Acid Deficiency

What may cause low omega-3-fatty acids? The following explanations may be some of the causes of a deficiency of this most important fatty acid.

- Alcoholism
- Carnitine deficiency
- Decreased intake of nutrients used as cofactors
- Excessive consumption of omega-6-fatty acids
- High intake of saturated fats
- Inability to absorb fatty acids
- Increased intake of sugar
- Increased intake of trans fatty acids
- Insufficient intake of dietary sources
- Stress
- Type I diabetes

■ Food Sources of Omega-3 Fatty Acids

Omega-3 is an essential fatty acid and it consists of four fatty acids: EPA, DHA, ALA, and DPA. The following are foods rich in each one of the acids.

Alpha-Linolenic Acid (ALA)

- Canola oil
- Dark green leafy vegetables
- Flaxseeds and flaxseed oil
- Hemp seeds and hemp oil
- Soybeans and soybean oil
- Tofu
- Walnuts and walnut oil

Docosahexaenoic Acid (DHA)

- DHA-enriched eggs
- Fatty fish, such as anchovies, herring, mackerel, salmon, sardines, and tuna
- Lamb
- Nuts

Eicosapentaenoic Acid (EPA)

- Fatty fish, such as anchovies, herring, mackerel, salmon, sardines, and tuna
- Lamb
- Nuts

Docosapentaenoic acid (DPA)

Docosapentaenoic acid (DPA) fish oil is a new omega-3-fatty acid that is sourced from a small, sustainable fish found in the Atlantic Ocean called menhaden which are lower on the food chain. This means that their oil is less likely to be filled with mercury and other toxins. DPA contains a higher concentration of omega-3-fatty acids than most other food sources.

Conditions That Can Benefit from Omega-3 Fatty Acids

There are not many nutrients as vital as omega-3 fatty acids and that is why it is referred to as an *essential* nutrient. This fatty acid is key and instrumental for your overall health, especially for conditions such as:

- Aggressive behavior
- Alzheimer's disease
- Arthritis (rheumatoid and degenerative)
- Asthma
- Atherogenesis
- Atopic dermatitis
- Attention-deficit/hyperactivity disorder (ADHD)
- Autism
- Bipolar disorder
- Cancer of the breast, colon, lung, prostate, and skin (prevention)
- Cardiovascular disease
- Cerebral palsy
- Chronic fatigue syndrome
- Coronary heart disease
- Crohn's disease
- Cystic fibrosis
- Depression
- Down syndrome
- Eczema

- Hypercholesterolemia (high cholesterol)

- Hypertension (high blood pressure)

- Hypertriglyceridemia (high triglycerides)

- Inflammation

- Irritable bowel syndrome (IBS)

- Macular degeneration

- Malignant cardiac arrhythmias (prevention)

- Migraine headaches

- Multiple sclerosis (MS)

- Neuropathy

- Polycystic ovarian syndrome (PCOS)

- Postpartum depression

- Premenstrual syndrome (PMS)

- Psoriasis

- Schizophrenia

- Stroke (prevention and recovery)

- Systemic lupus erythematosus (SLE)

- Type 2 diabetes (prevention and treatment)

- Weight loss

- Any other disease that has a significant inflammatory component

▓ Recommended Dosage

It is important that your intake of omega-6-fatty acids and omega-3-fatty acids maintain a proper ratio—between 3:1 and 6:1—or you may become deficient in omega-3s. This is because these two essential fatty acids compete for use in the body. Unfortunately, the standard American diet is very high in omega-6-fatty acids and very low in omega-3-fatty acids, so Americans (and most people worldwide) maintain a ratio of between 10:1 and 25:1. It is paramount that you eat foods that are high in omega-3-fatty acids, and you may need to take a supplement, as well.

The measurement of fatty acids is always the best way to determine the amount of fatty acids that you need. This test is available through several laboratories. (*See* Resources for contact information). You can also ask your healthcare provider to order a fatty acids test.

- General guidelines for adults under the age of 50: 1,000 milligrams a day

- General guidelines for adults over the age of 50: 2,000 milligrams a day

When you ingest omega-3-fatty acids, take vitamin E to prevent oxidation, a process that can result in damage from free radicals. To make sure that the fatty acids are converted into usable forms, also consume vitamin A, the B vitamins, vitamin C, biotin, magnesium, niacin, zinc, and protein. Omega-3 supplements can quickly oxidize and turn rancid. To prevent this, store your omega-3s in the refrigerator. If you find yourself "burping them up," try storing them in the freezer. This will not destroy their effectiveness.

■ Side Effects and Contraindications

In large doses, omega-3-fatty acids may act as a blood thinner, particularly in doses above 3,000 milligrams a day. Speak to your healthcare provider or pharmacist to learn if blood thinners or any other medications you're taking might make it unwise to use omega-3 supplements. The possible side effects associated with omega-3-fatty acids include: bad breath, belching, fishy taste, loose stools, nausea, and stomach upset.

Fish Oil vs Krill Oil Supplements

Both fish oil and krill oil supplements supply DHA and EPA, but there are differences. Krill oil comes from small crustaceans, not fatty fish, and typically contains more EPA. And unlike the omega-3s in conventional fish oil, krill oil's omega-3s are linked to an antioxidant and other potentially beneficial substances called phospholipids. Current research suggests that fish oil is beneficial for prevention and treatment of heart disease, and krill oil is a helpful therapy for arthritis and PMS.

LOW-DOSE NALTREXONE (LDN)

Naltrexone, a non-selective antagonist of opioid receptors, is mainly used as rehabilitation therapy for discharged opiate addicts to eliminate addiction in order to maintain a normal life and prevent or reduce relapse. In recent years, there have been some novel and significant findings on the off-label usage of naltrexone. It is hypothesized that lower than standard doses of naltrexone (low-dose naltrexone) inhibit cellular proliferation of T and B cells and block Toll-like receptor 4 (protein coding gene), resulting in an analgesic and anti-inflammatory effect. Low-dose naltrexone is a prescription compounded medication that very effectively reduces inflammation.

As you have seen, chronic inflammatory diseases are complex to treat and have an impact on a large number of individuals. Due to the difficulty of treating these diseases and the great impact on quality of life, patients often seek off-label, complimentary, or alternative medicines to gain relief from symptoms. Low-dose naltrexone (LDN) has been used off-label for treatment of pain and inflammation in many different diseases. Since COVID-19 has a large inflammatory component due to the manifestations of cytokine storm, LDN is now being used to treat COVID-19. Moreover, LDN can act as an immunomodulator in most autoimmune diseases and malignant tumors as well as alleviate the symptoms of some psychological disorders. LDN is also being effectively used for weight loss as well as prevention and treatment of memory loss.

The results of increasing studies indicate that LDN exerts its immunoregulatory activity by binding to opioid receptors in or on immune cells and tumor cells. Consequently, these new discoveries indicate that LDN may become a promising immunomodulatory agent in the therapy for cancer and many immune-related diseases.

Mechanisms of Action of LDN

Although LDN can be used for most autoimmune conditions, it is especially helpful for painful conditions due to its role in raising the level of endorphins in the body. LDN has also been shown to be beneficial for other conditions as well, since:

- LDN increases endogenous enkephalins and endorphins, which enhance immune function

- LDN inhibits pro-inflammatory cytokines, which improves the inflammatory reaction

- LDN interacts with the nuclear opioid growth factor receptor which promotes DNA synthesis

- LDN serves as a blockade of opiate-R in GI tract, which heals and repairs the mucosal tissue

- LDN regulates TReg and production of IL-10 and TGF-b, which down regulates TH-17

Side Effects

The following are potential short-term side effects of LDN:

- Fatigue
- Hair thinning
- Insomnia (the most common side effect)
- Loss of appetite
- Mild disorientation
- Mood swings
- Nausea
- Vivid dreams

There are also a few potential long-term side effects that may occur with LDN which include possible liver and kidney toxicity and potential tolerance to the beneficial effects. If you are taking a narcotic, you cannot take low dose naltrexone. Also, if you have acute hepatitis or liver failure then LDN is contraindicated.

LDN's Use in Treating Disease

New findings indicate that LDN is an encouraging immunomodulatory agent in the treatment of many immune-related diseases. LDN has been used for many different disease processes and conditions some of which are listed below.

- AIDS/HIV
- Amyotrophic lateral sclerosis (ALS)
- Atopic dermatitis
- Cancer
- Complex regional pain syndrome
- COVID-19
- Crohn's Disease
- Dry Eyes
- Eczema
- Fibromyalgia

- Herpes virus infections
- Irritable bowel syndrome
- Itching
- Lyme disease
- Multiple sclerosis
- Parkinson's disease
- Prevention/treatment of memory loss
- Psoriasis
- Rosacea
- Ulcerative colitis
- Weight loss

■ Recommended Dosage

Contact your healthcare provider to further discuss the use of LDN, which is a prescription. The dose is ramped up over time, commonly starting with 1.5 mg the first week, then 3 mg the second week and the 4.5 mg thereafter. Many dosage schedules of low-dose naltrexone are currently being used worldwide. It can also be given IV and used topically (transdermally).

CONCLUSION

As you have seen, the inflammatory response can be provoked by physical, chemical, and biologic agents, including mechanical trauma, exposure to excessive amounts of sunlight, x-rays and radioactive materials, corrosive chemicals, and temperature extremes. Furthermore, they can be provoked by infectious agents, such as bacteria, viruses, and other pathogenic microorganisms. Although these infectious agents can produce inflammation, infection and inflammation are not synonymous.

Remember, it is all about balance. A small amount of inflammation heals. Too much inflammation is linked to almost every major disease process including infections. The good news is that inflammation can be balanced using traditional medications, changing eating habits, adding nutrients and herbal therapies, and the newest anti-inflammatory drug therapy naltrexone (LDN) used at low doses. Low-dose naltrexone is one of the keys to the future of medicine for many disease processes that are inflammatory in nature.

9

Sleep
Get a Good Night's Sleep

Since the time of Hippocrates, the relationship between sleep and immunity has been the subject of discussion. A good night's sleep is paramount for proper functioning of your immune system.

Scientific evidence is building that sleep has powerful effects on immune functioning. Studies have shown that sleep loss can affect different parts of the immune system, which can lead to the development of a wide variety of diseases.

Trials have revealed that that if a person slept four hours a night it reduced their natural killer cell activity by about 72 percent, which increased their risk of developing viral infections and cancer. Furthermore, when individuals had reduced sleep, they exhibited an increase in the formation of inflammatory cytokines which are important in the development of many disorders, including immune system dysfunction.

In one study, sleep loss resulted in a greater than 50 percent decrease in the production of antibodies to influenza vaccination, in comparison with subjects who had regular sleep hours. In addition, with less sleep, people exhibit a decrease in antibody production, which increases their risk of common infection. Lastly, studies have also shown that not only do sleep-deprived people feel sleepy, but also other changes occur. Changes take place in their molecular, immune, and neural networks that play a role in the development of an exhaustive range of chronic health problems, such as obesity, diabetes, and cardiovascular disease.

One way to estimate your sleep-length need is to observe the length of time you sleep toward the end of a relaxing 2-week vacation, when you are not under time pressures and are sleeping freely (awakening spontaneously, without an alarm, and going to bed when you are tired). Keep caffeine intake to no more than 2 cups of regular coffee or tea a day. During the second week, record your bedtimes, wake-up times, and length of sleep. The average of the sleep times across the week is an estimate of your natural sleep-length need.

CIRCADIAN RHYTHM

The time frame in which you sleep is also significant. It is important to go to bed before 11:30 pm and not arise before 5 am otherwise the circadian rhythm in the body will change. Your circadian rhythm is a natural internal process that regulates your sleep-wake cycle.

Shift work is work done by an individual whose normal hours of work are outside the traditional 9 to 5 PM workday. It can involve evening or night shifts, early morning shifts, and rotating shifts which change the circadian rhythm in the body. It is common in many jobs, particularly those involving essential services. Shift workers represent between 15 percent and 25 percent of today's workforce in the world. Shift workers change the natural sleep rhythm of their body since work time poses a great challenge as it requires that they balance productivity and sleep time between shifts. Consequently, these employees experience chronic sleep deprivation with increases fatigue and drowsiness due to their sleep deprivation.

It is also of utmost importance to examine the fact that sleep and the circadian system exerts a strong regulatory influence on immune functions. Studies of the normal sleep–wake cycle showed that immune parameters, such as numbers of undifferentiated naive T cells and the production of pro-inflammatory cytokines, exhibit peaks during early nocturnal sleep. Whereas circulating numbers of cytotoxic natural killer cells, as well as anti-inflammatory cytokine activity cells peak during daytime wakefulness. Although it is difficult to separate the influence of sleep from that of the circadian rhythm, comparisons of the effects of sleeping at night with those of 24-hour periods of wakefulness suggest that sleep facilitates the discharge of T cells and their redistribution to lymph nodes. Moreover, studies reveal the enhancing influence of sleep on cytokines promoting the interaction between antigen presenting cells and T helper cells, like interleukin-12.

Furthermore, good sleep hygiene on the night after a vaccination was shown to produce a strong and persistent increase in the number of antigen-specific Th cells and antibody concentration. Together these findings represent a specific role of sleep in the formation of immunological memory. The endocrine environment during early sleep tends to promote the initiation of Th1 immune responses that eventually supports the formation of long-lasting immunological memories.

INSOMNIA

Insomnia is a common sleep disorder that is defined as difficulties with falling asleep, falling asleep but then awaking later, obtaining a deep sleep, and staying asleep throughout the night. Another key factor of insomnia is poor-quality sleep that does not alleviate fatigue in that you may experience non-restorative sleep. Regardless of how much sleep you get, if you have insomnia you seldom wake up feeling fresh and ready for the day. Non-restorative sleep may be classified by how long the symptoms are present. Temporary insomnia or transient insomnia, which is usually due to stress, lasts for less than a week, short term lasts from one to three weeks, and chronic insomnia or long-term may last for three weeks or more. Insomnia can drain not just your energy level and mood but also your health, job performance, and quality of life.

Insomnia is on the rise worldwide. An estimated 50 million to 70 million adults in the U.S. have chronic sleep and wakefulness disorders. These numbers are similar in other industrialized countries in proportion to the size of the country. Insomnia is more common in women (25 percent) than in men (18 percent), and its prevalence increases with age, affecting approximately 50 percent of elder people. Adequate sleep is foremost for your overall health, hormonal balance, and immune function.

Optimal hours of sleep are between $6^1/_2$ to 8 hours of sleep per night. Less than this time frame is not healthy and sleeping more than 8 hours a night is also not beneficial. Most people who say they do not need a great deal of sleep are pushing themselves to sleep less, and as a consequence, struggle to stay awake and function during the daytime. Long-term they are at risk for developing obesity and several other types of chronic illnesses.

SYMPTOMS OF INSOMNIA

Some indications of getting enough sleep are feeling refreshed after awakening and not being overly sleepy during the daytime. People who need several cups of regular coffee a day to feel alert may not be getting enough good-quality sleep. The following are common symptoms of insomnia:

- Concerns about sleep
- Daytime tiredness or sleepiness
- Difficulty falling asleep at night
- Difficulty focusing or paying attention
- Early morning awakening
- Increased errors
- Increased risk of being in an accident
- Irritability, depression, or anxiety

- Memory lapses
- Not feeling well-rested after a night's sleep
- Waking up during the night

CAUSES OF INSOMNIA

The causes of insomnia depend on whether it is primary or secondary insomnia. Primary insomnia is *not* associated with a medical or psychiatric illness. Secondary insomnia, which is most common, is a symptom of a fundamental disorder, such as illness, stress, anxiety, hormonal imbalance, or depression that may resolve with treatment of the disease process. Furthermore, insomnia may be a trigger for other disease processes, such as epilepsy.

Chronic insomnia is usually a result of stress, life events, or habits that disrupt sleep. Treating the underlying cause can resolve the insomnia, but sometimes it can last for years.

Concerns about your job, school, finances, family, death of loved one, or illness may keep your mind active and lead to insomnia. A disruption in your circadian system, poor sleep habits, such irregular bedtimes, stimulating activities, using your bed for work, or eating too much too late can lead to wakeful nights.

Caffeinated drinks and alcohol may be causes of insomnia as well. Caffeine acts as a stimulant and when consumed in the late afternoon or evening it can prevent you from falling asleep. Alcohol may make it easier for you to fall asleep at the onset, but it can interfere with deeper stages of sleep and may cause you to wake up in the middle of the night.

Some medications may interfere with sleep. Discontinuing or changing medications may be beneficial to help with insomnia. If you are taking one of these medications and have insomnia, do not discontinue the medication without discussing this with your healthcare provider. Commonly your doctor, physician's assistant, nurse clinician, or pharmacists may suggest another medication that will aid in treating your disease process that may not cause insomnia as a side effect. The following are some of the medications that may disrupt sleep or cause insomnia.

- ACE inhibitors
- Alpha blockers
- Angiotensin receptor blockers (ARBs)
- Antiarrhythmics
- Anticonvulsants
- Antihistamines
- Appetite suppressants
- Benzodiazepines (tranquilizers)
- Beta blockers

- Bronchodilators
- Carbidopa/Levodopa
- Cholinesterase inhibitors
- Corticosteroids
- Diuretics (water pills)
- Decongestants
- Estrogen without progesterone to balance
- Lipophilic beta blockers
- Medication that contains caffeine

- Monoamine oxidase inhibitors
- Nicotine
- Pseudoephedrine
- Selective serotonin reuptake inhibitors (SSRIs)
- Sedatives
- Statin drugs
- Sympathomimetics
- Tetrahydrozoline
- Thyroid hormones
- Tricyclic antidepressants

CONVENTIONAL THERAPIES

Since chronic insomnia can last for a long time and can seriously affect one's well-being and quality of life, many people turn to conventional medications to find relief. The following are traditional medications that have been used to treat insomnia. Traditionally insomnia is treated by classical hypnotics, such as benzodiazepines and Z drugs (this class includes zolpidem, zopiclone, zaleplon, and eszopiclone), which both act on the GABA-A receptor. Potentially, they may have many side effects, including cognitive impairment, tolerance, rebound insomnia upon discontinuation, increase in car accidents and falls, abuse, and drug dependence.

Newer medications for insomnia, such as melatonergic agonist drugs, agomelatine, prolonged-release melatonin, ramelteon, and tasimelteon, are now being used more commonly.

Innovative drugs that have recently come on the market target the orexin/hypocretin system. They potentially have fewer side effects in terms of drug-drug interactions, interactions with alcohol, less memory impairment, and dependence potential compared to classical hypnotics.

In addition, there is some evidence for the use of the quetiapine, trazodone, mirtazapine, amitriptyline, pregabalin, gabapentin, agomelatine, and olanzapine as treatments for insomnia. These drugs may improve sleep while successfully treating comorbid disorders, disorders existing simultaneously, with a different side effect profile than the older medications. Other modalities, such as non-drug therapies and cognitive behavioral therapy, have also been traditionally recommended.

PERSONALIZED MEDICINE THERAPIES

Conventionally, medications and cognitive behavioral therapy have been used to treat primary or secondary insomnia without looking at the etiology of the disease process itself. The following review examines the causes of the insomnia as part of the treatment of this common disorder along with other therapies.

Diet

The right diet is an important part of the journey in curing insomnia. In creating a diet for insomnia, you need to avoid foods that could make it worse and consume foods that could make it better. It is important to avoid processed foods with preservatives and avoid all foods with stimulant properties.

A study revealed that a Mediterranean-style diet was associated with adequate sleep duration, less insomnia symptoms, and the participants were less likely to have insomnia accompanied by short sleep. Likewise, a low intake of vegetables and fish and a higher intake of sugary foods and pasta were independently associated with poor sleep quality in another trial.

Poor sleep quality was also associated with high carbohydrate intake in free-living Japanese middle-aged female workers. Reactive hypoglycemia (sugar crash within four hours of eating a high carbohydrate meal) has been shown to be an etiology of insomnia. Eat more frequent healthy meals. Complex carbohydrates—such as lentils, lima beans, and peas—have been shown to help you fall asleep, since they protect your blood sugar from highs and lows.

If you commonly consume foods that you have an allergic response to, you may experience insomnia due to an elevation of epinephrine and norepinephrine that occurs when you eat these types of foods. Allergy testing may be helpful since many allergies are sensitivities (IgG responses) and not true food allergies (IgE responses). The severity of symptoms ranges from mild to life-threatening. Generally, however, a food allergy will result in one or more of the following physical responses:

- Abdominal pain
- Anal itching
- Anaphylaxis
- Anemia
- Anxiety
- Backache
- Breathing difficulties
- Cancer sores
- Chest pain
- Cracks at the corners of your mouth
- Dark circles under your eyes

- Diarrhea
- Eczema
- Fatigue
- Fluid retention
- Food cravings
- Frequent urination
- Gas
- Headaches
- Heart palpitations
- Heartburn
- Hives
- Hoarseness
- Itchy, watery eyes
- Itchy skin

- Low blood pressure
- Muscle aches
- Nasal congestion
- Nausea
- Persistent cough
- Rash
- Reddened earlobes, eyes, or cheeks
- Ringing in ears (tinnitus)
- Sniffling and sneezing
- Stomach cramps
- Tension headaches
- Tremors
- Wrinkling under eyes

Likewise, foods that contain stimulant properties cause the body to work harder to carry out the digestive process and removal of toxins from the body. These include:

- Aspartame. Insomnia has been reported by individuals to be a side effect of aspartame use. Try stopping artificial sweeteners if you are using them.

- Caffeine. Some people, particular ones that are slow acetylators, have insomnia due to caffeine intake. Do not drink more than two 8-oz beverages that contain caffeine a day and finish them by noon.

- Excessive sodium. Eating a meal that is high in salt at dinner time, or after dinner, can contribute to sleep disturbances due to a rise in blood pressure and fluid retention. High sodium foods abound and include less obvious foods, such as pickles, olives, cheese, and pizza.

- Sugar. Sugar, especially refined sugar, is known to disrupt your blood glucose levels, creating highs and lows that affect your whole nervous system.

Exercise

Exercise is important for your body and mind, and it can also aid in getting a good night's sleep. Nevertheless, you need to be mindful of the timing. For some, exercising too late in the day can interfere with how well they rest at night.

A study revealed that exercise was beneficial to decrease sleep complaints. In fact, exercise provided similar results when compared with hypnotics —a sleep-inducing drug. Another study examined workers, particularly sedentary older workers, having sleep problems reported less high-intensity leisure-time physical activity. This data suggests that a vicious circle may indeed prevail between poor sleep and reduced leisure-time physical activity.

Exercise can be invigorating and may keep you awake. Change your exercise routine to the morning and see if this is helpful. In addition, higher body temperatures also interfere with sleep. This is another reason to exercise at least 4 hours prior to bedtime.

Electronics

Cell phones, tablets, computers and other electronic devices have become such an enormous part of everyday life that it is often hard to put them down producing poor sleep patterns. Your phone, TV, or computer may be the reason you're suffering from sleeplessness.

There's now little reservation among scientists that a relationship exists between screen exposure at night and sleep quality. The results of a study showed that computer usage for playing/surfing/reading was positively associated with insomnia, and negatively associated with being most active and alert during the morning. Likewise, mobile phone usage for playing/surfing/texting was positively associated with insomnia and chronotype (one's propensity for sleep at a specific time in a 24-hour period) and negatively associated with being a morning person.

The blue light released by screens on cell phones, computers, tablets, and televisions decreases the production of melatonin, the hormone that regulates your sleep/wake cycle or circadian rhythm. Lowering melatonin levels makes it harder to fall and stay asleep.

Hormones

Insomnia can also be related to a hormone imbalance. A hormone disparity can result in sleep problems, and a lack of sleep can cause further hormonal imbalances. The following are hormone imbalances that may cause your sleeplessness:

- **Testosterone.** In a male, low testosterone levels may be associated with insomnia. Consequently, testosterone replacement may be an effective therapy for insomnia. See your doctor and have your testosterone level measured. It is also important to understand that large doses of exogenous testosterone and anabolic/androgenic steroid (synthetic testosterone) abuse are associated with abnormalities of sleep duration and architecture. In addition, several studies have reported that sleep loss can lower testosterone levels in the body.

Reports of decreased testosterone following one night of total sleep deprivation have varied from 18.5 percent to 30.4 percent decreases in plasma testosterone, and a 27 percent decrease in salivary testosterone. Sleep restriction has shown similar, yet smaller, effects of sleep loss on testosterone. When sleeping only the first half of the night for eight nights, men experienced a 10 to 15 percent reduction in testosterone as evidence in a medical trial.

- **Estrogen.** As a result of hormonal imbalances, women experience insomnia at just about twice the rate of men. Low estrogen levels commonly result in insomnia. Women suffering from insomnia related to vasomotor symptoms (VMS)—night sweats, hot flashes, and flushes—can be effectively treated with natural hormone replacement therapy (BHRT). In addition, natural estrogen replacement therapy, in menopausal and postmenopausal women, has been shown to improve sleep by decreasing night-time awakenings.

- **Progesterone.** Studies also revealed that decreases in progesterone levels can cause disturbed sleep. Progesterone has both sedative and anti-anxiety effects, stimulating benzodiazepine receptors, which play an important role in the sleep cycle.

- **DHEA and Cortisol.** Underlying mechanisms show that stress is involved in the relationship between sleep and metabolism through hypothalamic–pituitary–adrenal (HPA) axis activation. Sleep deprivation and sleep disorders are associated with maladaptive changes in the HPA axis, leading to neuroendocrine dysregulation. Hormonal balance is a key component for sleep regulation. See your healthcare provider or pharmacist for salivary hormone testing of your sex hormones, as well as DHEA and cortisol.

- **Melatonin.** Melatonin regulates sleep, in addition, this hormone has many other functions, such as:

  - Acts as an antioxidant
  - Affects the release of sex hormones
  - Aids in stroke prevention and treatment

  - Aids the immune system
  - Blocks estrogen from binding to receptor sites
  - Decreases cortisol levels and helps balance the stress response

- Decreases inflammation (lowers c-reactive protein and Il-6)
- Free radical scavenger
- Heart protective due to its vasodilating actions
- Helps prevent and treat memory loss
- Helps prevent cancer
- Improves mood
- Improves sleep quality
- Lowers blood pressure
- Protects against reflux
- Stimulates the parathyroid gland
- Stimulates the production of growth hormone

Melatonin levels gradually decrease with aging and may be linked to lowered sleep efficacy.

If you eat too many high glycemic index carbohydrates, you will make less melatonin. Melatonin levels can also be lowered by excessive intake of alcohol and caffeine. Tobacco use can decrease melatonin levels as can electro-magnetic fields.

Melatonin supplementation induces drowsiness and sleep, and may ameliorate sleep disturbances, including the nocturnal awakenings associated with the aging process. Always have your melatonin level measured by saliva testing and replace according to lab levels. If you take too much melatonin it may lower serotonin, your neurotransmitter that contributes to feelings of happiness.

- **Insulin.** Insulin is a vital hormone that is naturally manufactured by the body and directs cells in the body to remove glucose from the blood and use it for energy. Scientists have discovered that insulin resistance (a condition in which cells fail to normally respond to insulin) is closely linked to loss of sleep. Insulin levels tend to rise if you do not have good sleep hygiene. A study revealed that sleep restriction (5 hours a night) for one week significantly reduced insulin sensitivity. Therefore, raising concerns about effects of chronic insufficient sleep on disease processes associated with insulin resistance and diabetes.

Neurotransmitters

Neurotransmitters are chemical messengers in the body. Their function is to send signals from nerve cells to target cells. These target cells include muscles, glands, or other nerves. The brain calls for neurotransmitters to regulate many essential functions, one being sleep cycles. The neurotransmitters connected with driving wakefulness and sleep include histamine, dopamine, norepinephrine, serotonin, glutamate, and acetylcholine.

Depending on the time of day one makes these neurotransmitters, they can keep us focused and alert or prohibit sleep and cause wakefulness. In fact, they have a clinical effect on the "clock" that is responsible for keeping our circadian rhythm in check. For instance, serotonin is a calming neurotransmitter, and if your levels of it are too low, it can result in sleep problems.

- **L-tryptophan.** L-tryptophan is a neurotransmitter that is a precursor to serotonin, which plays a major role in sleep hygiene, helping to create healthy sleeping patterns as well as elevating your mood. Some studies have shown that L-tryptophan is helpful and some trials do not show it to be of benefit. Furthermore, do not use L-tryptophan if you are on an anti-depressant unless you are under the direct supervision of your doctor. Ask your healthcare provider or pharmacist to order a neurotransmitter test to determine optimal dosage.

  DOSE: 1 to 2 grams 30 to 60 minutes before bedtime, on an empty stomach with a small amount of carbohydrate. This dose is for people with normal renal function. Also consider taking niacin, vitamin B6, and magnesium along with the tryptophan to increase its conversion into serotonin.

- **5-HTP.** 5-HTP is closer to serotonin in the pathway and does not need a transport system to carry it into the brain. Several studies have shown 5-HTP to be effective; perhaps more effective than L-tryptophan in treating insomnia since it increases REM sleep. Ask your healthcare provider or pharmacist to order a neurotransmitter test to determine optimal dosage.

  DOSE: The usual suggested dosage is 100 to 300 mg taken 30 to 60 minutes before bedtime. It is recommended that you start with 100 mg. If you are taking an anti-depressant, do not use L-tryptophan or 5-HTP without consulting your healthcare provider.

Nutrients

In addition to medications and lifestyle changes, there are several nutrients and vitamins that may be therapeutic for insomnia and provide quality sleep. Studies indicate that some vitamins may improve your sleep. They include:

- **Vitamin B12** has been shown to be helpful in some people but not others for insomnia. Vitamin B12 deficiency is common in older people. Vitamin B12 takes part in the production of melatonin and is therefore necessary for quality sleep.

  DOSE: Recommended dosage for an adult is 1,000 micrograms.

- **Niacinamide,** a supplemental form of niacin, when taken at bedtime depresses the central nervous system which helps you fall asleep and stay asleep.

  DOSE: Niacinamide at 1,000 mg at night may be beneficial.

In addition to vitamins, other nutrients are also vital for quality sleep, such as:

- **Magnesium** taken one hour before bedtime may be helpful since one of the symptoms of low magnesium is insomnia. Magnesium increases blood melatonin levels, which help to improve your quality of sleep. Magnesium has also been shown to be helpful for restless leg syndrome which is one of the causes of insomnia.

  DOSE: A double-blind study showed that giving 250 mg of magnesium twice a day helped with sleep in patients that had moderate to severe insomnia. Another suggested dosage is 400 mg of magnesium glycinate one hour before bedtime to help with poor sleep hygiene.

- **L-theanine** promotes relaxation and sleep by increasing levels of GABA as well as serotonin and dopamine; calming brain chemicals produced by the body. Studies have shown L-theanine to be beneficial for sleep. Since it can affect neurotransmitter balance, it is suggested to have neurotransmitter testing performed.

  DOSE: Recommended dosage is 100 to 200 mg twice a day. L-theanine needs to be taken twice a day in order for it to work for insomnia. L-theanine is an amino acid that is found in both black and green tea.

Herbal Therapies

Herbs have been used in the treatment of insomnia for more than 2000 years. According to scientific research, insomnia has been effectively treated by herbal formulas. Herbs recognized as effective sleep remedies include:

- **Valarian** (*Valeriana officinalis*)—a tall flowering grassland plant—has been shown in double-blind studies to decrease sleep onset latency and improve the quality of sleep. It should be taken 30 minutes to one hour before bedtime. Some individuals experience morning sleepiness the next day.

- **Hops** (*Humulus lupulus*)—flowers of the hop plant—is a beneficial herbal therapy for insomnia. Although Hops shows promise for alleviating anxiety and sleep disorders on their own, they might be increasingly effective when combined with valerian. The German Commission E has listed Hops as an approved therapy for insomnia.

- **Lemon balm** (*Melissa officinalis*) can be used along or in combination with other herbal therapies for insomnia particularly in menopausal women. Combination formulas of both Lemon balm and Valerian have been shown to be effective.

  DOSE: 300 to 500 mg capsules of dried leaf. This herb should not be used by women that are pregnant or lactating. This herb is from the mint family. Do not use if you are allergic to mint.

CONCLUSION

In summary, chronic sleep deprivation can be seen as an unspecific state of chronic stress, which negatively impacts immune functions and your health in general. The adverse effects of long-term sleep deprivation comprise an enhanced risk for various diseases as a consequence of a persistent low-grade systemic inflammation on the one hand, as well as immunodeficiency characterized by an enhanced susceptibility to infections and a reduced immune response to vaccination on the other hand. Getting enough sleep is crucial to your overall health in many ways; from positively affecting cortisol levels in your body to dramatically enhancing your immune system.

10

Smoking
How It Affects the Immune System

More than 400,000 people die each year in the United States alone as a result of past or current cigarette smoke use. In addition, adult smokers lose an average 13 to 15 years of life-expectancy because they smoke. Despite widespread knowledge of the risks posed by smoking, the worldwide prevalence of tobacco use is estimated to be more than one billion people. Cigarette smoking is considered the most preventable cause of death in developed nations.

Therefore, smoking is one of the major lifestyle factors influencing your health. Life-long cigarette smokers have a higher prevalence of common diseases, such as heart disease and chronic obstructive pulmonary disorder (COPD). Long-term smoke exposure can result in increased products of lipid peroxidation—resulting in cell damage—and decreased levels of antioxidants, such as vitamins A and C, in the blood of smokers. Inflammatory markers, such as c-reactive protein (CRP), fibrinogen, and interleukin-6 (IL-6), are elevated in long-term smokers as well as an increased white blood cell (WBC) count may be present. Furthermore, coagulation and endothelial function (regulation of inflammation in tissues) markers are altered in chronic cigarette smokers. PAI-1 (Plasminogen activator inhibitor-1) levels that are elevated increase your risk of thrombosis (clotting) and atherosclerosis. A deficiency of PAI-1 causes abnormal bleeding. This marker also plays an important role in adhesion, migration, cell proliferation, and signal transduction pathways.

SYSTEMS AFFECTED BY CIGARETTE SMOKE

Smoking tobacco has various effects on your body systems. It affects the respiratory system, the circulatory system, the reproductive system, the skin, and the eyes, and it increases the risk of many different cancers. The main affected system by cigarette smoke is the respiratory tract. In bronchial epithelium metaplastic (abnormal change of lung tissue) and dysplastic (abnormal growth) changes are accompanied by elevated expression of adhesion molecules and secretion of many cytokines capable of stimulation immune cells influx. Likewise, pulmonary macrophages experience changes in surface markers with impaired phagocytic—cells capable of absorbing bacteria—and antigen function. Macrophages are the most numerous immune cells present in the lung environment. Moreover, chronic exposure to cigarette smoke causes increased production of enzymes causing destruction of the alveolar wall of the lung.

Furthermore, cigarette smoke causes diverse changes in immunity that lead to heightened constitutive inflammation, skewing of adaptive T cell-mediated immunity, impaired responses to pathogens, and suppressed anti-tumor immune cell functions. When the exposure to cigarette smoke is long-term, a chronic inflammatory process develops that has the potential to promote enhanced microbial colonization and infection, persistence of apoptotic (programmed cell death) material, abnormal processing of cellular debris, induction of autoimmunity (where the immune system reacts against the body's own components), and architectural remodeling.

Although most of smoking-induced changes are reversible after quitting, some inflammatory mediators like CRP (c-reactive protein) are still significantly elevated in ex-smokers up to 10 to 20 years after quitting. This suggests a low-grade inflammatory response persisting in former smokers long-term. In addition, many immunological changes in smokers are not completely reversible after they quit smoking.

HARMFUL CONTENTS OF TOBACCO SMOKE

Cigarette tobacco is made from dried tobacco leaves, and other materials are added for flavor to make smoking desirable. This tobacco smoke created from these products is a complex mixture of chemicals made by burning tobacco and its additives. Nicotine, which is one of the main constituents of cigarette smoke, suppresses the immune system according to clinical trials. In addition, cigarette smoke is known to increase susceptibility to infections and certain cancers.

Both natural killer cells (NK) and interleukin (IL)-15 play crucial roles in innate immunity against viral infections and cancer, and they are impaired by the chemicals released from tobacco smoke. In addition, interleukin-15 plays an important role in immune responses by regulating proliferation, survival, and functions of NK cells. The influence of tobacco smoke on human health is still an important problem worldwide.

Cigarette smoking has a negative effect on your health due to what is in the tobacco smoke. It is not just nicotine. Dr. Grant Cooper in his book, *Never Smoke Again*, lists the following as just a fraction of the harmful contents that are found in cigarette smoke.

- Acetone
- Arsenic
- Benzene
- Butadiene (a flammable hydrocarbon)
- Carbon monoxide
- Cyanide
- DDT (insecticide)
- Dieldrin (hazardous chemical used in insecticides)
- Formaldehyde
- Lead
- Naphthalene (used to make mothballs)
- Styrene (used to make Styrofoam)
- Vinyl chloride

NICOTINE ADDICTION

Nicotine, a highly addictive chemical, is both physically and psychologically habit-forming. Cigarette smoke is physically addictive since habitual users come to crave the chemical and mentally addictive given that users knowingly desire the effects of nicotine. Most people go through withdrawal symptoms when they try to quit smoking. You may experience some, but probably not all of these if you are trying to quit smoking.

- Anxiety
- Constipation
- Cough
- Cravings
- Depression
- Difficulty concentrating
- Dizziness
- Dry mouth
- Fatigue
- Headache
- Hunger
- Insomnia
- Irritability
- Postnasal drip
- Sore throat

TREATMENTS TO HELP YOU BREAK THE HABIT

A number of treatments are available to help you quit smoking by getting you past your craving for nicotine. These include both conventional therapies, including behavioral support, and personalized medicine therapies.

Conventional Therapies

Since the development of nicotine replacement therapy (NRT) in 1978, treatment options have continued to evolve and expand to aid individuals in smoking cessation. Despite this, currently available treatments remain insufficient, with less than 25 percent of smokers remaining abstinent one year after treatment. The two main approaches to assist cessation are pharmacotherapy and behavioral support.

Pharmacotherapy

Pharmacotherapy for smoking cessation aims primarily to reduce the intensity of urges to smoke and/or ameliorate the aversive symptoms. These are all prescription medications and may cause significant side effects in some individuals. They also may interact with other medications. Make sure that you have a long discussion concerning the pros and cons of each of these medications before starting drug therapy.

- **Varenicline** is generally considered the most effective drug available for treatment of tobacco dependence. It decreases both cravings and the pleasurable effects of nicotine addiction. Possible mild side effects include: constipation, gas, insomnia, usual dreams, changes in taste, headache, nausea, and vomiting. Serious side effects may also occur.

- **Bupropion** has also been shown to be effective as a first-line drug. In one randomized, double-blind trail, smoking cessation rates after 6 months were 35 percent with bupropion alone and almost 40 percent with bupropion plus nicotine. The drug's most common negative effects are insomnia and dry mouth. Other side effects may include: anxiety, agitation, stuffy nose, stomach pain, shakiness, nausea, nervousness, loss of appetite, headache, drowsiness, dizziness, diarrhea, and constipation. Serious side effects can also transpire.

- **Clonidine** and **nortriptyline** are second-line treatments used when first-line treatments fail or are contraindicated, or by patient preference. Although second-line drugs have been shown to be effective, their use is limited due to a less favorable side-effect profile compared to the first-line therapies previously discussed.

- **Memantine, baclofen, topiramate, galantamine**, and **bromocriptine** may be used if other therapies have failed.

- **Nicotine replacement therapy** has been shown to be effective in some individuals but has a higher side effect profile than any other form of treatment.

Nicotine is available as a prescription patch, gum, lozenge, nasal spray, and inhaler depending on the state and country that you live in.

Behavioral Support

Behavioral support aims to boost motivation to resist the urge to smoke and develop a person's capacity to employ their plans to avoid smoking. These interventions usually last only a few months. The goal is thought that during these months, the strength of the associative learning between smoking and reward diminishes and most symptoms of withdrawal remit. After these few months, most smokers should have overcome their addiction and should be able to remain off cigarettes. Hypnosis has also been shown to be effective for some individuals. Furthermore, a good exercise program may be helpful since it serves as both a distraction as well as a form of meditation. Exercise also has a positive effect on mood.

Studies have shown that a combination of both a behavioral and pharmacological approach is more effective in smoking cessation than either approach alone.

Personalized Medicine Therapies

Personalized medicine therapies have also been shown to be beneficial for some patients, including:

- Novel therapies such as n-acetyl cysteine (NAC) are displaying promising results. N-acetyl cysteine has antioxidant properties, both increasing glutathione and modulating glutamatergic, neurotropic, mitochondrial, and inflammatory pathways. It is well tolerated, with a side effect profile that does not differ significantly from placebo in clinical trials when given orally at doses up to 3 grams a day, the exception being mild gastrointestinal side effects. NAC may also improve some of the physical harms caused by tobacco smoke exposure, improving mucociliary transport, which is the self-clearing mechanism of the airways in the respiratory system. NAC also prevents oxidative damage to the lungs and other tissues. See Part 3 of this book for a further discussion of NAC.

- Studies have found that people who smoke, and those who are exposed to secondhand smoke, have reduced amounts of vitamin C in their bodies. Smokers should take an additional 2,000 mg of vitamin C a day.

- Tai chi, acupuncture, yoga, hypnotherapy, and mindfulness meditation have also been shown to be helpful.

CONCLUSION

If you smoke: find a way to quit! When you begin, it appears as if it is a long road, however after a few weeks it starts to feel like a hazy memory. It can seem daunting and unbearable at times, but using the suggestions in this chapter, you can get through it. If you give up your smoking habit while you are healthy, your body can heal from most, or all, of the damage done by smoking. The rewards and benefits are worth it.

11

Stress
Manage Your Stress

We all deal with stress at some point in our lives. Your experiencing stress when your body reacts to pressure from certain situations. It can be your job, a family issue, illness, or money troubles. Your immune system is inherently related to your stress levels. Stress is an all-encompassing concept that comprises both challenging circumstances that are stressful along with both the psychological and physical response to stress. One of the major systems in the body that reacts to demanding circumstances is the immune system. In fact, numerous facets of the immune system are associated with stress. This chapter will explore the concept of stress and how you can mitigate this important key to health. A small amount of stress keeps you on your toes, a large amount of stress causes distress to the body.

ACUTE/CHRONIC STRESS

Acute stress is when your feel stressed for a short period of time. However when you are first stressed within minutes, the body prepares for injury or infection during what is called a "flight or fight" response. It also increases blood levels of pro-inflammatory cytokines. Research has revealed that short-term stress boosted the immune system.

Likewise, long-term stress—chronic stress—lasts for months or even years and furthermore, it is associated with elevated levels of inflammatory cytokines, but it has different consequences. Initially the body produces an inflammatory response to help the body heal and help the body eliminate pathogens. However, long-term inflammation causes dysregulation of the immune system and increases your risk of developing many other diseases, which are further discussed in the section on inflammation, page 96. In addition, another consequence of chronic stress is initiation of latent viruses. Latent virus activation can reflect the loss of immunological control over the virus and frequent activation can cause wear-and-tear on the immune system.

Interestingly, these responses may not be the same for all individuals. Early life stressors can compromise the immune system. In addition, as people age, they are less able to mount an appropriate immune response to stressors that are both physical and psychological. Studies have suggested that older adults are unable to terminate cortisol production in response to stress. Chronic elevations of cortisol can lead to the immune system becoming "resistant," with an accumulation of stress hormones, and increased production of inflammatory cytokines that further compromises the immune response.

HOW DOES STRESS INFLUENCE IMMUNITY?

Immune cells have receptors for neurotransmitters and hormones, such as norepinephrine, epinephrine, and cortisol. They mobilize and traffic immune cells, that prepare the body to mount an immune response if needed. Recent trials have shown that immunological cells (for example, lymphocytes) change their responsiveness to signaling from these neurotransmitters and hormones during stress. Likewise, immunological responses expend energy and over time deplete the body of some of its energy stores. Consequently, chronic stress produces negative systemic changes in the immune system and the remainder of the body.

Other potential mediators, like getting a good night's sleep, are progressively being recognized as important pieces of the stress-immunity continuum. Even one night of total sleep deprivation was recently found to significantly increase neutrophil counts and decrease neutrophil function in healthy males. For further information, *see* chapter 9 on good sleep hygiene and the immune system.

In other words, when you are stressed and you stay stressed, your immune system becomes compromised. Furthermore, the cumulative effect of daily stressors promotes elevations in inflammatory markers.

CORTISOL

Your body makes a hormone named cortisol which is also called the "stress hormone" due to its involvement in your response to stress. Cortisol is the only hormone in your body that increases with age. Chronic stress has been shown to contribute to accelerated aging and premature death in medical studies. One study suggested that as many as 75 percent to 90 percent of visits to primary care doctors are stress related.

Cortisol is made in the adrenal glands and is derived from pregnenolone. Cortisol levels are regulated by adrenocorticotropic hormone (ACTH), which is synthesized by the pituitary in response to corticotropin-releasing hormone (CRH). CRH is produced by the hypothalamus which is located in the brain.

Prolonged activation of the stress-response process and the overexposure to cortisol and other stress hormones will potentially play havoc with almost all your body's systems. Retaining the right cortisol balance is key for human health, and you can experience setbacks if you produce too much or too little cortisol. For example:

• Low levels of cortisol: hypocortisolism, hypoadrenalism, adrenal fatigue

• High levels of cortisol: hypercortisolism, hyperadrenalism

• Lack of cortisol production: Addison's disease

• Very excessive cortisol production: Cushing's disease

Cortisol has quite a few essential functions in the body. In fact, if your body stops making cortisol, you pass away within a week. In other words, the making of cortisol is essential for life. It also plays an important role in a number of tasks your body carries out. For example, it:

• Aids in sleep

• Anti-inflammatory

• Balances blood sugar

• Balances DHEA

• Controls weight

• Helps with protein synthesis

• Improves mood and thoughts

• Participates with aldosterone in sodium reabsorption

• Regulates bone turnover rate

• Regulates immune system response

• Regulates the stress response

When you are stressed, cortisol levels elevate. As stress decreases, the levels go back down and normalize. However, in contemporary culture, most people are stressed all the time. Overbooking is an issue with almost everyone. If you have too many tasks on your plate or you multitask frequently, your body will remain in a state of constant stress. One of the most important things that you can do to control your stress is to gain control of your time. In addition, one of the main stresses in today's world is that many people are worried whether their immune system is functioning optimally. This puts a unique stress on the body, consequently cortisol levels remain abnormal, which further compromises the immune response.

ELEVATED LEVELS OF CORTISOL

While cortisol frequently gets a bad name, it's really crucial for your health and survival. It's only a concern if your cortisol levels are elevated for a prolonged period of time. An increased cortisol level can be indicative of several things discussed in this chapter, the worst of which is Cushing's syndrome. Physically, Cushing syndrome produces a fatty lump between the shoulders, an appearance of a rounded face, and purple or pink stretch marks on the skin. Cushing's syndrome can also lead to high blood pressure, weight gain, acne, thin skin, easy bruising, muscle weakness, bone loss, and injuries that are slow to heal. Other symptoms of Cushing's syndrome include mood swings, irritability, depression, and anxiety. Some individuals also experience a headache and have an increased incidence of infection.

Causes of Elevated Cortisol Levels

The following are other causes of elevated cortisol levels:

- Chronic pain
- Depression
- Excessive alcohol intake
- Excessive sugar intake
- Exposure to toxins
- Hypoglycemia (low blood sugar)
- Infections
- Inflammation
- Oral contraceptives
- Poor sleep hygiene
- Stress
- Weight gain

■ Signs and Symptoms of Elevated Cortisol Levels

The signs and symptoms of elevated cortisol levels differ according to what is causing the increase in your cortisol levels. They may include:

- Binge eating
- Compromised immune system
  - Decrease in antibody release
  - Increase in infection rate
  - Increase in the release of inflammatory cytokines
  - Inhibition of the proliferation of T cells
- Inhibition of the release of some cytokines
- Latent (delayed) virus activation
- Shift from Th1 to Th2 cytokine expression
- Confusion
- Easy bruising
- Elevated blood pressure

- Fatigue
- Impaired hepatic conversion of T4 to T3 (which causes the thyroid gland not to work as well)
- Increase in:
  - Blood sugar/insulin resistance/diabetes
  - Cholesterol
  - Development of leaky gut syndrome (increase in intestinal permeability)
  - Osteoporosis risk by causing loss of minerals in the bones

- Triglycerides
- Irritability
- Low energy
- Memory is not as sharp
- Muscle weakness
- Night sweats
- Shakiness between meals
- Sleep disturbances
- Sugar cravings
- Thin skin
- Weight gain around the middle

PERSONALIZED MEDICINE THERAPIES TO LOWER ELEVATED CORTISOL LEVELS

The following therapies are in the order they should be considered for elevated cortisol levels. Begin with stress reduction techniques. Prayer, meditation, tai chi, yoga, chi gong, breathing exercises, exercise (not strenuous), music, dancing, and acupuncture have all been shown to be beneficial. Figure out what works for you when you feel your stress levels rising. Stress can be harnessed to fuel success and achievement. However, if your stress is to the point of "distress," then this is problematic. You may want to consider:

- Nutrients containing:
  - B vitamins
  - Calcium
  - Copper
  - Magnesium
  - Manganese
  - Selenium
  - Sodium
  - Vitamin C
  - Zinc
- Adaptogenic herbs:

- Ashwagandha
- Cordyceps sinensis
- Ginkgo biloba
- Panax ginseng
- Rhodiola rosea
- Calming herbs, if needed, such as lavender, passionflower, lemon balm, and chamomile
- If cortisol is high in the evening, then add phosphatidylserine 300 mg which may be taken anytime of the day.

CORTISOL DEFICIENCY

Long-term stress depletes the body of cortisol and eventually you only make enough cortisol to stay alive. You must have cortisol to live. Your body, therefore, goes into a state of emergency when you stay stressed for many months or even years. You may not feel well. You may turn to coffee, tea, soft drinks, or sugar as a source of energy, but this will only make the situation worse. Consuming any of these items will temporarily make you feel better or more energetic, but the negative effects far outweigh the temporary fix.

If your adrenal glands stay stimulated, they may weaken and "burn out." When this happens, your cortisol and DHEA levels will drop. This is called adrenal fatigue, hypocortisolism, or hypoadrenalism. If the adrenal glands become totally depleted, it is called Addison's disease. This is a medical emergency. If you have Addison's your body does not make any cortisol at all. Adrenal fatigue is not a total depletion of cortisol, but it does bring cortisol levels down low enough to prevent optimal functioning of the body. Adrenal fatigue is one of the most pervasive and under-diagnosed syndromes of modern society.

■ Signs and Symptoms of Cortisol Deficiency (Adrenal Fatigue)

The appearance of cortisol deficiency can be associated with any of the following signs and/or symptoms listed below.

- Allergies (environmental sensitivities and chemical intolerances)
- Decreased immunity
- Decreased sexual interest
- Digestive problems
- Emotional imbalances
- Emotional paralysis
- Fatigue
- Feeling of being overwhelmed
- General feeling of "un-wellness"
- Hypoglycemia
- Increased PCOS, PMS, peri-menopause, and menopausal symptoms
- Increased risk of alcoholism and drug addiction
- Increased symptoms of andropause
- Lack of stamina
- Loss of motivation or initiative
- Low blood pressure
- Poor healing of wounds
- Progressively poorer athletic performance
- Sensitivity to light

- Unresponsive hypothyroidism (low thyroid function that does not respond to thyroid replacement)

Causes of Cortisol Deficiency

Cortisol is fundamental to proper function of many of the body's systems. The circumstances that trigger inadequate levels of cortisol to be produced can happen for various reasons, such as:

- Chronic inflammation
- Chronic pain
- Depression
- Dysbiosis (bacteria in your gastrointestinal tract become unbalanced)
- Hypoglycemia (low blood sugar)
- Long-term stress
- Nutritional deficiencies
- Overly aggressive exercise
- Poor sleep hygiene
- Severe allergies
- Toxic exposure

PERSONALIZED MEDICINE THERAPIES TO RAISE CORTISOL

The following therapies are in the order they should be considered for low cortisol levels. Begin with stress reduction techniques. Prayer, meditation, tai chi, yoga, chi gong, breathing exercises, exercise (not strenuous), music, dancing, and acupuncture have all been shown to be beneficial. Running a hot bath and curling up with a good book are all effective ways to reduce stress.

- Nutrients containing:
  - B vitamins
  - Vitamin C
  - Calcium
  - Copper
  - Magnesium
  - Manganese
  - Selenium
  - Sodium
  - Zinc
- Adaptogenic herbs:
  - Ashwagandha
- Cordyceps sinensis
- Panax ginseng
- Rhodiola rosea
- Calming herbs, if needed, such as lavender, passionflower, lemon balm, and chamomile
- Adrenal extracts (if adaptogenic herbs do not work)
- Licorice (the herb)
  - It cannot be used if you have hypertension (high blood pressure).

- If you develop hypertension while taking it, then discontinue the licorice.
- Cortef
  - It is a last resort therapy. This means that all of the above therapies have been tried first. It is a steroid prescription drug that is used to augment the cortisol in your body and should not be used to replace cortisol.
  - Cortef is only to be used for six to nine months. Continue adrenal extract with the cortef so when your healthcare provider weans you off cortef your stress hormone stabilizes. If the cortisol level becomes elevated, then stop the adrenal extracts and restart the adaptogenic herbs.

Usually, it takes six months of constant stress or more for adrenal fatigue to settle in. However, once you start treatment for your exhausted adrenal glands, it takes one to two years or even longer for your glands to heal completely.

CONDITIONS ASSOCIATED WITH ABNORMAL LEVELS OF CORTISOL

Abnormal cortisol levels that are too high or too low can be associated with many medical conditions including a compromised immune system.

- Accelerates the aging process by advancing cellular aging and shortening telomere length
- Alzheimer's disease/other forms of cognitive decline
- Andropause (male menopause)
- Anorexia nervosa
- Anxiety disorders
- Breast cancer
- Chronic fatigue syndrome
- Coronary heart disease
- Depression
- Fibromyalgia
- Impotence
- Infertility
- Insulin resistance/diabetes
- Irritable bowel syndrome (IBS)
- Menopause
- Multiple sclerosis
- Osteopenia/osteoporosis
- Panic disorders
- Polycystic ovary syndrome (PCOS)
- Post-traumatic stress disorder (PTSD)
- Premenstrual syndrome (PMS)
- Rheumatoid arthritis
- Sleep disorder

CONCLUSION

Research concerning the stress hormone cortisol has shown the large toll that both acute and chronic stress has on the immune system. In addition, studies concerning the effects of stress on inflammation have demonstrated that chronic stress can increase the likelihood of the development of many different disease processes, as well as exacerbating preexisting conditions. Therefore, it is paramount that you have your cortisol levels evaluated.

Optimal measure of cortisol for the purpose of evaluating the stress response, and not for the diagnosis of Addison's disease or Cushing's disease, is via salivary testing. Testing for cortisol levels will not be accurate if you have been on steroids within the last 30 days.

Furthermore, many individuals with abnormal cortisol levels also have a thyroid that is not functioning to its full potential (hypothyroidism). It is important to always work on fixing the adrenal glands before thyroid medication is instituted; otherwise, the symptoms of depleted or elevated cortisol levels may be made worse. *See* chapter 13 on thyroid hormone and the immune system.

12

Sugar
Minimize Your Intake
for Healthy Eating

E ating healthy is essential to a healthy existence and well-being. Consuming healthy food helps you to sustain a healthy weight and decrease your risk of type 2 diabetes, high blood pressure, high cholesterol, and the threat of developing cardiovascular disease, as well as several forms of cancer. There are many healthy eating programs available for people to partake in. However, the scope of this chapter is not to discuss all the programs that are available but to encourage healthy eating. There is one item that every person would benefit from in a healthy eating program: minimize your sugar intake.

Cutting back on the amount of sugar in your diet can help you reduce the risk of the health conditions cited above. Substituting high sugar foods with healthful choices can help you obtain all of the essential vitamins and minerals needed by your body, minus the additional calories. It may also help with weight loss.

SUGAR

Foods with *sugars added* make for extra calories in your diet but contribute little *nutritional value*. Refined sugar is 99.4 percent to 99.7 percent pure calories. There are no vitamins, minerals, or proteins. It is just carbohydrates. The body needs chromium, manganese, cobalt, copper, zinc, and magnesium to digest sugar. These minerals have been stripped from the sugar during the refining process. Consequently, the body depletes its own mineral reserves to process the sugar.

Predominantly, people are able to recognize desserts and candy as having added sugar, but how about the less obvious sources? Foods that most people would believe to be "healthy" may surprisingly have a lot of added sugar in them. There are hidden sugars in food that many people are not aware of. Just because the labels claim the product is "whole grain" or "fortified with vitamins and minerals," such as breakfast cereals, doesn't mean there's no sugar. In addition, some ketchups are one-half sugar, peanut butter may have sugar added, and sugar may be added to hamburgers sold in restaurants to decrease shrinkage.

Sugar comes in many forms, some of which are not as easily recognizable.

- Agave syrup or nectar
- Barley malt
- Beet sugar
- Brown sugar
- Cane sugar
- Cane syrup
- Confectioners' sugar
- Crystalline fructose
- Date sugar
- Evaporated sugarcane
- Fructose
- Fruit juice or concentrate
- Galactose
- Glucose
- Granulated sugar
- High fructose corn syrup
- Honey
- Invert sugar
- Lactose
- Liquid cane sugar or syrup
- Maltose (malt sugar)
- Maple syrup
- Molasses
- Powdered sugar
- Raw sugar
- Rice syrup
- Sugarcane syrup
- Table sugar
- Turbinado sugar
- Unrefined sugar
- White sugar

Reasons Why Sugar Can Harm Your Health

An excess of added sugar in your diet can result in many negative health effects. Numerous major authors have examined this idea in the past. Dr. Nancy Appleton has explored the idea of sugar and its relationship to almost every major illness there is in her book *Suicide by Sugar*. Dr. Appleton spent 20 years collecting reasons why sugar can ruin your health. The following is a summary of the list developed by Dr. Appleton. Note the first item on her list: *Sugar can suppress the immune system.*

- Sugar can suppress the immune system.

- Sugar upsets the mineral relationships in the body.

- Sugar can increase reactive oxygen species (ROS), which damage cells and tissues.

- Sugar can cause hyperactivity, anxiety, inability to concentrate, and crankiness in children.

- Sugar can produce a significant rise in triglycerides, lower HDL (good cholesterol), and raise LDL (bad cholesterol).

- Sugar causes a decline in tissue elasticity and function; the more sugar you eat the more elasticity and function you lose.

- Sugar intake that is high can increase the risk of developing several different forms of cancer.

- Sugar can raise blood sugar and increase the risk of developing insulin resistance and diabetes.

- Sugar increases the risk of developing cataracts.

- Sugar increases the risk of developing macular degeneration.

- Sugar raises the levels of the neurotransmitters: dopamine, serotonin, and norepinephrine.

- Sugar can lead to tooth decay and salivary acidity.

- Sugar can cause premature aging by lowering growth hormone, the hormone that keeps you young.

- Sugar causes inflammation.

- Sugar can lead to an acidic digestive tract.

- Sugar can lead to weight gain and obesity.

- Sugar increases the risk of developing Crohn's disease and ulcerative colitis.

- Sugar increases the risk of developing arthritis.

- Sugar increases the risk of developing gastric and duodenal ulcers.

- Sugar assists the uncontrolled growth of Candida albicans (yeast infections).

- Sugar can cause gallstones.

- Sugar increases the risk of developing heart disease.

- Sugar increases the risk of developing appendicitis.

- Sugar increases the risk of developing varicose veins.

- Sugar increases the risk of developing osteoporosis (bone loss).

- Sugar contributes to food allergies.

- Sugar can impair the structure of DNA and change the structure of protein.

- Sugar can contribute to emphysema and asthma.

- Sugar can interfere with the absorption of protein.

- Sugar increases advanced glycation end products (AGEs).

- Sugar can cause the skin the wrinkle by changing the structure of collagen.

- Sugar can contribute to fatty liver.

- Sugar can damage the pancreas.

- Sugar can cause fluid retention.

- Sugar slows food's travel time through the gastrointestinal tract and can increase the number of bowel movements.

- Sugar can increase the risk of developing headaches including migraine.

- Sugar can increase the risk of developing gout.

- Sugar can contribute to myopia (nearsightedness).

- Sugar can contribute to all forms of memory loss.

- Sugar increases the risk of developing kidney stones.

- Sugar can cause free radicals and oxidative stress.

- Sugar contributes to hormonal imbalances of insulin, thyroid, adrenal hormones DHEA and cortisol, and also the sex hormones estrogen, progesterone, testosterone.

- Sugar is addictive.

- Sugar can cause decrease emotional stability by causing moodiness nervousness, anxiety, and depression.

- Sugar promotes excessive food intake in overweight and obese people.

- Sugar can worsen ADD/ADHD.

- Sugar can contribute to seizures.

- Sugar can cause constipation.

- Sugar increases the risk of developing metabolic syndrome.

- Sugar increases the risk of developing irritable bowel syndrome.

- Sugar contributes to acne.

- Sugar can contribute to the development of diverticulitis.

- Sugar can make essential nutrients less available to cells.

- Sugar can increase uric acid in the blood and increase the risk of developing gout.

- Sugar can cause hypoglycemia.

SUGAR SUBSTITUTES

Trying to minimize the sugar and calories in your diet? You may be resorting to artificial sweeteners or other sugar substitutes if you cannot have sugar. These sugar substitutes are food additives and they are equivalent to the taste of sugar however have less food energy. Artificial sweeteners and other sugar substitutes are found in a range of foods and beverages advertised as "sugar-free" or "diet," including soft drinks and baked goods. What are all these sugar substitutes found in foods and what role do they play in your diet? Let's examine each of the sugar substitutes.

Aspartame. Aspartame, a non-saccharide artificial sweetener, is 200 times sweeter than sugar. Once your body processes aspartame, a portion of it is broken down into methanol. Methanol is toxic in sizable amounts, yet smaller quantities may also be worrisome. Since 2014, aspartame has been identified as the predominate source of methanol in the American diet. Research has recognized a link between aspartame and a host of conditions which may have any of these possible following side effects.

- ADD/ADHD
- Altered gut microbiota
- Disorientation
- Dizziness
- Ear buzzing
- Elevated cortisol
- Elevated liver enzymes (SGOT)
- Eye hemorrhages
- Gut dysbiosis by altering
- Headaches

- High blood pressure
- Hives
- Inflammation of the pancreas
- Loss of equilibrium
- Memory loss
- Numbness of extremities
- Seizures
- Severe muscle aches
- Tunnel vision
- Visual impairment

Sucralose. Sucralose starts with a sugar molecule and has three of its components removed and replaced with chloride. It provides no calories because the body does not recognize it as a food. Sucralose does not raise blood sugar but is 2,000 times sweeter than sugar. As of the FDA's approval in 1998, studies have surfaced about sucralose's possible negative side effects. The risks of consuming large quantities of sucralose may include diabetes, cancer, weight gain, and gastric issues. In addition, it may increase the development of hypothyroidism, since chloride may replace iodine in the body when using a lot of sucralose. Iodine is needed for optimal thyroid function. It is also an antibacterial, anticancer, antiparasitic, antiviral, and mucolytic agent.

Honey. Honey contains small amounts of vitamins and minerals and is 20 percent to 60 percent sweeter than sugar. The primary argument behind the negative effect of consuming too much honey is the excessive amount of fructose existing in honey. This high proportion of fructose in honey diminishes the ability of the small intestine to metabolize nutrients appropriately.

Saccharin. Saccharin, one of the oldest artificial sweeteners, has been used for over 100 years. Limited research exists on the side effects of saccharin, however, a possible link may exist between consuming saccharin in substantial amounts and high blood sugar and alterations in gut bacteria.

Stevia. Stevia is extracted from a leaf and has no known side effects. It does not raise glucose or insulin (the hormone that regulates blood sugar) levels in the body.

Sugar alcohols. Sugar alcohols are naturally occurring sweet compounds found in fruits and vegetables. Supplements are made from the fiber of birth trees. Sugar alcohols include: xylitol, sorbitol, mannitol, and isomalt. They may decrease the incidence of dental cavities. They fight plaque buildup and neutralize plaque acids. Sugar alcohols also increase satiety. They have 40 percent less calories than sugar and have a minimal effect on blood sugar and insulin levels. The body produces up to 15 grams of xylitol per day from other food sources. Sugar alcohols are incompletely absorbed in the intestine and may have a laxative effect, especially if used in large quantities.

Other artificial sweeteners that are currently permitted in the United States and other countries include, acesulfame potassium, neotame and advantame, which are both similar to aspartame, and luo han guo fruit extract. Refined sugars (for example, sucrose, fructose) were absent in the diet of most people until very recently in history.

SUGAR ADDICTION

Overconsumption of sugar-rich foods or beverages is initially motivated by the pleasure of sweet taste and is often compared to drug addiction in medical studies. One medical trial revealed that intense sweetness can surpass cocaine reward, even in drug-sensitized and addicted individuals. Sugar has been shown to activate opiate receptors in the brain, which affects the reward center, leading to compulsive behavior even though the individual knows that eating too much sugar may cause weight gain and have other negative affects upon the body.

In addition, excessive sugar intake causes an increase in the release dopamine, a neurotransmitter, which gives a person the feeling of a "high" and makes an individual want to repeat the behavior. Likewise, the appetite for sugar is propelled by shifts in the hunger-satiety progression which facilitates cravings for sugar in the absence of energy needs. In other words, in both animals and human studies, substantial commonalities are exhibited between drugs of abuse and sugar, from the standpoint of brain neurochemistry as well as behavior.

REACTIVE HYPOGLYCEMIA

Your blood sugar levels fluctuate throughout the day, the levels go up and down. When the sugar or glucose levels in your blood measure too low, it can result in a condition called hypoglycemia. As insulin (the hormone that regulates blood sugar) levels elevate, glucose drops which results in reactive hypoglycemia. This condition refers to an occurrence of hypoglycemia in no more than four hours following a high carbohydrate meal. Additional potential causes of reactive hypoglycemia include alcohol consumption, certain surgical procedures (gastric bypass or surgery for an ulcer), inherited metabolic disorders, and various tumors.

■ Symptoms of Reactive Hypoglycemia

The symptoms of reactive hypoglycemia usually occur not long after you eat. Signs and symptoms can include:

- Abdominal pains/gas/diarrhea
- Blurred vision
- Cramps in the feet and legs
- Dizziness, light-headedness

- Faintness/fainting
- Feeling sleepy/drugged
- Flushing/sweating
- Impaired memory

- Insomnia
- Mental confusion/inability to concentrate
- Nervousness, depression, irritability
- Numbness or tingling in the hands, feet, or face
- Overwhelming fatigue
- Palpitations, irregular heartbeat
- Pressure in the head/frontal headache
- Ringing in the ears
- Severe anxiety/panic attacks
- Trembling of the hands
- Sensation of butterflies in the stomach

To manage reactive hypoglycemia, eat smaller, more frequent meals to help restore a higher blood sugar level. In addition, you need to include lots of lean protein and complex carbs in your diet, as they are slower to digest, which helps control your blood sugar levels.

CONCLUSION

Long-term use of added sugar can be a problem for many people and can result in numerous medical conditions. Sugar upsets the balance of all the systems in the body, especially the immune system. Like many things in life, moderation is the key to health. It is all about balance. Sweet snacking is a frequent behavior at times of stress. Find another method of stress reduction. Remember: *Stressed* spelled backwards is *desserts*!

13

Thyroid
Optimize Its Function

Documentation accumulated over recent decades has revealed a connection between thyroid hormones and the immune system. Thyroid hormone metabolism and thyroid status have been linked to various aspects of the immune response. Changes in the levels of thyroid hormones can notably affect the activity of the immune system and play crucial roles in both the innate and adaptive immune responses. Thyroid hormones can influence the responses in various immune cells—monocytes, macrophages, natural killer cells, and lymphocytes.

An overactive thyroid (hyperthyroidism) causes your systems to function too fast, whereas, an underactive thyroid (hypothyroidism) causes your systems to perform too slowly. One possible explanation for thyroid problems is an impaired immune system. This chapter will focus on hypothyroidism.

HYPOTHYROIDISM

Hypothyroidism is defined as low thyroid function, or an underactive thyroid, where the thyroid gland does not make enough thyroid hormones to allow the body to function optimally. The main function of the thyroid hormone is to oversee your metabolism; therefore, people with this condition have symptoms associated with a low functioning metabolism. Hypothyroidism disturbs the normal equilibrium of the chemical reactions in the body.

Hypothyroidism is a more common disorder than you may think. About 27 million Americans suffer from either an overactive or underactive thyroid gland and over 200 million people have a thyroid disorder. Of these, around 80 percent of them are women. People of any age can suffer from hypothyroidism, but it is more common in older adults. A woman is five to eight times more inclined to have an underactive thyroid than a man, and women over the age of 50 are at a higher risk. While hypothyroidism can take several forms, the most common is Hashimoto's thyroiditis which is an autoimmune process where the body is being intolerant of the antigens on its own cells.

SIGNS AND SYMPTOMS OF HYPOTHYROIDISM

Unfortunately, the earliest signs and symptoms of low thyroid function can occur several years prior to laboratory results being abnormal. It is therefore important to be aware of this disorder's signs and symptoms including an immune system that is not functioning at its peak performance.

The following are signs and symptoms of hypothyroidism.

- Acne
- Agitation/irritability
- Allergies
- Anxiety/panic attacks
- Arrhythmias (irregular heartbeat)
- Arthralgias/joint stiffness
- Bladder and kidney infections
- Blepharospasm (eye twitches)
- Brittle, ridged, striated, thickened nails
- Carpel tunnel syndrome
- Cognitive decline
- Cold hands and feet
- Cold intolerance
- Congestive heart failure
- Constipation
- Coronary heart disease/acute myocardial infarction (heart attack)
- Decreased cardiac output
- Decreased sexual interest
- Delayed deep tendon reflexes
- Deposition of mucin in connective tissues
- Depression
- Dizziness/vertigo
- Down turned mouth
- Drooping eyelids
- Dull facial expression
- Ear canal that is dry, scaly, and may itch
- Easily broken nails
- Easy bruising
- Eating disorders
- Elbow keratosis (rough, scaly skin)
- Endometriosis
- Erectile dysfunction
- Excess formation of cerumen (ear wax) in the ear canal
- Fatigue
- "Fat pads" above the clavicles
- Fibrocystic breast disease
- Fluid retention
- Gallstones

- Hair loss in the front and back of the head
- Headaches, including migraine headaches
- High cortisol levels
- High c-reactive protein (CRP)
- Hoarse, husky voice
- Hypercholesterolemia
- Hyperhomocysteinemia (high homocysteine levels)
- Hyperinsulinemia (high insulin levels)
- Hypertension
- Hypoglycemia (low blood sugar)
- Impaired kidney function
- Inability to concentrate
- Increased appetite
- Increased risk of developing asthma
- Increased risk of developing bipolar disorder
- Increased risk of developing schizoid or affective psychoses
- Infertility
- Insomnia
- Iron deficiency anemia
- Loss of eyelashes, or eyelashes that are not as thick
- Loss of hair in varying amounts from legs, axilla, and arms
- Loss of one-third of the eyebrows ("Queen Anne's sign)

- Low amplitude theta and delta waves on EEG
- Low blood pressure
- Low body temperature
- Menorrhagia (abnormally heavy and prolonged menstrual cycle)
- Menstrual irregularities
- Mild elevation of liver enzymes
- Miscarriage
- Morning stiffness
- Muscle and joint pain
- Muscle cramps
- Muscle weakness
- Myxedema
- Nocturia (need to get up in the middle of the night and urinate)
- Nutritional imbalances
- Osteopenia/osteoporosis (bone loss)
- Painful menstrual cycles
- Paresthesias (prickling, burning, tingling, numb, itching, or "skin crawling" feeling)
- Poor circulation
- Poor night vision
- Premenstrual syndrome (PMS)
- Puffy face
- Reduced heart rate
- Rough, dry skin
- Shortness of breath
- Sleep apnea
- Slow movements

- Slow speech
- Sparse, coarse, dry hair
- Swollen eyelids
- Swollen legs, feet, hands, and abdomen
- Tendency to develop allergies

- Tinnitus (ringing in the ears)
- Vitamin B12 deficiency
- Weight gain
- Yellowish discoloration of the skin due to the inability to convert beta carotene into vitamin A

THYROID HORMONES

The body makes more than one kind of thyroid hormone, as well, as TSH which is thyroid stimulating hormone. They are:

- Diiodothyronine (T2)
- Triiodothyronine (T3)
- Thyroxine (T4)
- Reverse triiodothyronine (rT3)

T4 Production and Conversion of T4 to T3

If you have a thyroid disorder, such as hypothyroidism, you may be tested to assess how well your body is producing and converting T4, the main thyroid hormone, to T3, the more active thyroid hormone. Deficiencies of zinc, copper, vitamins A, B2, B3, B6, and C are factors that cause decreased production of T4. Furthermore, in order for thyroid function to be optimal, your body must easily convert T4 to T3 in order to use it. The conversion of T4 to T3 requires the enzyme 5'deiodinase. There are three types of 5'deiodinases.

1. Type I is located in the thyroid, liver, and kidney and plays an important role in the production of T3

2. Type II is found in the pituitary, hypothalamus, and brown fat and converts T4 to T3

3. Type III catalyzes deiodination—removal of iodine—of the inner ring of T4 to T3, which inactivates the hormone

Production of 5'Deiodinase

The following elements affect the production of 5'deiodinase:

- Cadmium, mercury, and lead toxicity
- Chronic illness
- Decreased kidney or liver function
- Elevated cortisol

- High carbohydrate diet
- Inadequate protein intake
- Inflammation

- Selenium deficiency
- Starvation
- Stress

Conversion of T4 to T3

There are many factors that affect the conversion of T4 to the more active T3.

Nutritional deficiencies:

- Iron
- Selenium
- T3 Iodine

- Vitamins A, B2, B6, and B12
- Zinc

Medications:

- Amiodarone
- Beta blockers (such as propranolol)
- Clomipramine
- Estrogen replacement
- Glucocorticoids
- Interleukin (IL-6)

- Lithium
- Oral contraceptives
- Phenytoin
- Propylthiouracil
- Some chemotherapeutic agents
- Theophylline

Diet:

- Eating too many walnuts
- Excessive alcohol use
- Low carbohydrate diet
- Low fat diet

- Low protein diet
- Too many cruciferous vegetables (broccoli, cauliflower, kale, Brussels sprouts)
- Soy

Other Factors:

- Aging process
- Calcium excess
- Copper excess
- Diabetes
- Dioxins
- Fluoride

- GI infections
- High dose alpha lipoic acid (600 mg and above)
- Inadequate production DHEA and/or cortisol
- Lead toxicity

- Lyme disease
- Mercury
- PCBs
- Pesticides
- Phthalates (chemicals added to plastics)
- Radiation
- Stress
- Surgery
- Toxic mold syndrome
- Viral infections

Low T3 or Increased Reverse T3

The following are factors that are associated with low T3 or increased reverse T3.

- Aging process
- Diabetes
- Elevated levels of IL-6, TNF-alpha, IFN-2
- Fasting
- Free radical production
- Increased levels of epinephrine and/or norepinephrine
- Prolonged illness
- Stress
- Toxic metal exposure

Nutrients to Increase Conversion of T4 to T3

Fortunately, there are substances that can increase the conversion of T4 to T3.

- Ashwagandha (an herb)
- Glucagon (a hormone that is involved in blood sugar control)
- Growth hormone replacement
- High protein diet
- Insulin
- Iodine
- Iron
- Melatonin
- Potassium
- Replacement of testosterone in men (decreases the concentration of thyroid binding globulin)
- Selenium
- Tyrosine (an amino acid)
- Vitamins A, B2, E
- Zinc

EVALUATING YOUR THYROID FUNCTION

It is very important that when you see your healthcare provider for evaluation of your thyroid gland that you have complete blood work done and not partial testing. The following studies are paramount to be evaluated in order to determine if you have low thyroid function. It is also key that you have optimal levels of thyroid hormone and not just normal levels.

The following are a list of the complete panel of thyroid hormones that you should have done and also the optimal range of thyroid hormone for each lab.

TABLE13.1 OPTIMAL RANGE OF THYROID HORMONES	
Thyroid Hormone	Optimal Range
TSH (thyroid stimulating hormone)	0.3–5.5 (optimal is 0.3 to 2.0 uU/mL)
Free T3	Mid-range of normal
Free T4	Mid-range of normal
Reverse T3	Within normal range
Thyroid antibodies: —Antithyroglobulin antibody —Anti-microsomal antibody —Anti-thyroperoxidase antibody (anti-TPO)	Al three antibodies within normal range

Some people will have normal or even optimal levels of thyroid hormone but still will have symptoms of hypothyroidism. For these individuals it is important to get a basal body temperature. A basal body temperature is the temperature underneath your arm taken before you get out of bed in the morning for ten minutes. You take your temperature for three consecutive days. If you are a menstruating woman, then take your temperature during your menstrual cycle.

Thyroid binding globulin (TBG) can also be measured. This is the amount of stored hormone. It is produced by the liver and is affected by illness, liver disease, and some medications. Sometimes estrogens can raise TBG so this is another test that you doctor may order.

Your healthcare provider may also order thyroid releasing hormone (TRH) also called thyrotropin-releasing factor (TRF) which is a hormone that stimulates the release of thyroid stimulating hormone (TSH) and prolactin from the pituitary.

Some patients have an autoimmune process where their body is literally trying to attack its own thyroid gland and the body produces a normal amount of thyroid hormone or not enough thyroid hormone. This is called Hashimoto's thyroiditis, where your test results reveal that your thyroid antibody levels are high.

TREATMENT OF HYPOTHYROIDISM

There are several things to consider in looking at treatment for low thyroid function. You may benefit from detoxification of the liver or helping your gut to be healthy. You may have nutritional deficiencies and improving your nutritional status may improve your thyroid function. You may be taking a medication that causes your thyroid not to function as well as it could. This does not mean that you should stop your medication, but it does mean that certain medications may affect thyroid function. In that case, you may have to replace a nutrient that is depleted due to the medication or you may have to take thyroid medication due to another drug that you are taking. Lastly, you may benefit from thyroid replacement as a medication.

Detoxification

Sometimes individuals with hypothyroidism do not need medication but would benefit from detoxification. Before embarking upon a detox plan, you want to make certain you have eliminated the source of toxicity. You cannot repair the damage until you have removed the source. PCBs, dioxins, DDT, HCB (hexachlorobenzene), phthalates, and high levels of heavy metals, such lead, arsenic, and mercury, can also cause dysfunction of your thyroid gland. Watch out for environmental toxins that target thyroid hormone receptors. It is possible to measure levels of most of these toxins and then have them removed. Sometimes when your GI tract health is improved by using the 5R program (*see* chapter 7) you may no longer have symptoms of hypothyroidism and the labs also normalize.

Nutritional Therapies

Medications are not always needed to improve thyroid performance. If you are deficient in basic nutrients, then starting a multivitamin may help your thyroid function improve. In addition, various vitamins and minerals can act as an effective underactive thyroid therapy. Two essential nutrients that are frequently deficient when a thyroid disorder exists are selenium and iodine. Consider having levels of iodine and selenium measured by your healthcare provider to see if you have an optimal supply of these important nutrients.

Other nutrients are also important for thyroid function, including iron magnesium, B vitamins, vitamin D, and zinc.

Iodine

According to the World Health Organization, up to 72 percent of the world's population is affected by an iodine deficiency disorder. Iodine deficiency is a major cause of hypothyroidism. Iodine has therapeutic actions in the body. It is an antibacterial, anticancer, antiparasitic, antiviral, and mucolytic agent. The thyroid gland uses iodine on a daily basis. Other organs in the body use iodine besides the thyroid gland: breast, prostate, kidneys, spleen, liver, blood, salivary glands, and intestines all use iodine. There are many causes of iodine deficiency including the following:

- Diet that is high in pasta and breads which contain bromide (bromide binds to iodine receptors and prevents iodine from binding)

- Diets without ocean fish or sea vegetables such as seaweed

- Fluoride use (inhibits iodine binding)

- Ground your food is grown in is deplete in iodine

- Inadequate use of iodized salt (low salt diet) in a region (Midwest), which is low in iodine

- Ipratropium nasal spray (contains bromide)

- Medications that contains bromide or fluoride can lead to iodine deficiency. Listed below are some examples.
  - Atrovent inhaler (contains bromide)
  - Flonase (contains fluoride)
  - Flovent (contains fluoride)

- Sucralose (artificial sweetener that contains chlorinated table sugar)

- Vegan and vegetarian diets

Iodine is needed for the production of thyroid hormones. The U.S. Institute of Medicine recommends a daily intake of 150 micrograms to 290 micrograms of iodine. The upper of normal recommended daily is 1,100 micrograms in an adult.

Many conditions beside hypothyroidism may be improved with iodine supplementation including:

- Dupuytren's contracture

- Excess mucous production

- Fatigue

- Fibrocystic breast disease

- Headaches and migraine headaches

- Hemorrhoids

- Keloids

- Ovarian cysts

- Parotid duct stones

- Peyronie's disease

- Sebaceous cysts

Breast health is related to iodine levels. Studies have shown that areas of the world with high iodine intake like Japan have a lower rate of breast cancer. It is estimated that the breasts need approximately 5 mg of iodine per day in a 50 kg woman.

If you are allergic to shellfish, then you should not take iodine as a supplement. If you take thyroid hormone and you then start taking iodine you may need less thyroid medication. Therefore, it is best if you have your iodine levels measured before you start on thyroid hormone. In fact, sometimes your symptoms of hypothyroidism may resolve and your labs may normalize with just taking iodine, if you are low in this important nutrient. Most people do better when they take iodine supplements to take both iodine and iodide as one preparation.

You can get too much of a good thing. Consequently, it is very important that you have your iodine levels measured before you start taking iodine. Too much iodine in the diet, or by supplementation, has been associated with thyroiditis, which is an inflammation of your thyroid gland. Elevated levels of iodine can cause iodine to be trapped by thyroglobulin. Raised levels of iodinated thyroglobulin then prompt the immune system to react and to cause inflammation. Furthermore, research has shown that in some areas of the world where there is high dietary iodine content or excessive supplementation, there is also an increase in not just thyroiditis but also thyroid cancer. Therefore, it is paramount that you have your iodine levels measured before you begin iodine replacement.

If you have already started thyroid medication and do not feel better, then it is still suggested to have your iodine levels measured. Urinary iodine testing is the gold standard. After you have started an iodine supplement, then your levels should be re-measured again in three to six months.

Selenium

Many people are aware that iodine is crucial to thyroid health. Selenium is less prominent but equally as important. Selenium is a vital nutrient for the body and nowhere is this more noticeable than the thyroid. In order for the thyroid to perform optimally, it must obtain the proper nutrition, and that means getting enough selenium. In the absence of this important mineral, thyroid hormone metabolism is impaired given that iodine-based enzymes cannot be composed, and these enzymes are essential for the activation of thyroid hormones. Your body does not synthesize its own selenium. Therefore, all selenium needs to be obtained through food or supplements. Selenium also boosts your immune system by increasing the effectiveness of white blood cells which help to ward off infections.

Iron

In order for your thyroid to function optimally you also have to have enough iron in your body. Optimal levels of ferritin (iron) are 100 ng/ml. If you are a cycling woman then your ferritin levels should be at least 130 ng/ml, since you lose iron every menstrual cycle. High levels of ferritin increase your risk of heart disease, so ask your healthcare provider if you need to take iron. In addition, iron is necessary for optimal immune system health.

Magnesium

Magnesium is an important supplement since most people are deficient in this mineral. Seven out of every ten Americans suffer from magnesium deficiency. Although there are several symptoms resulting from magnesium deficiency, the most common one is low thyroid function. Magnesium is necessary for the proper absorption of iodine. In addition, although magnesium is essential to every organ in your body, it is particularly important in the function of the heart, kidneys, and muscles.

Magnesium deficiency can result when you take large doses of vitamin C. The problem being that vitamin C competes with magnesium. Furthermore, healthy thyroid function relies on a balance of calcium and magnesium in the body. Other causes of magnesium deficiency include:

- Alcohol abuse
- Certain medications
- Diarrhea
- Eating a diet high in trans fatty acids
- Excessive sugar intake
- Extreme athletic competition
- Gastrointestinal disorders
- High caffeine intake
- High consumption of foods and drinks high in oxalic acid (such as almonds, cocoa, spinach, and tea)
- Minimal intake of foods rich in magnesium
- Phosphates in soft drinks
- Poor absorption
- Stress
- Surgery
- Taking magnesium supplements while eating a high fiber meal
- Trauma

B Vitamins

A deficiency in vitamin B2 can contribute to a low functioning thyroid. A lack of Vitamin B2 suppresses the production of T4 and the thyroid and adrenal glands from secreting their hormones. Vitamin B3 is needed to keep the endocrine cells in efficient working order. It plays a role in the production of thyroid hormones. Vitamin B3 is needed to produce tyrosine (an amino acid) in the body, and T3 and T4 are derived from tyrosine. Also, be aware that taking vitamin B2 (riboflavin) and vitamin B3 (niacin) is crucial if you are on iodine supplementation. It is also important in maintaining a healthy thyroid.

Vitamin D

Like magnesium, many people are not aware that they have low levels of vitamin D. Low levels of vitamin D may interfere with the thyroid functioning properly. Everyone can benefit from having their vitamin D levels measured, particularly if you have an autoimmune disease. The relationship between Hashimoto's thyroiditis and vitamin D has been demonstrated in several studies. Vitamin D deficiency is frequent in Hashimoto's thyroiditis. Treatment of patients with this disease with vitamin D may slow down the course of development of hypothyroidism and decrease the risk of heart disease. You can request your vitamin D level to be checked when you have your next blood test with your healthcare provider. Besides taking daily vitamin D supplements, daily exposure to sun is beneficial to your overall well-being.

Zinc

Zinc is a trace mineral, which is required for the synthesis of thyroid hormones. Without the existence of zinc in the body the thyroid cannot convert the inactive hormone T4 to the active hormone T3. The hypothalamus also depends upon zinc to make the hormone it uses to cue the pituitary gland to switch on the thyroid. Too little zinc leads to a low functioning thyroid. In fact, zinc is a cofactor in over 100 reactions in the body. Chronic zinc deficiency can weaken your immune system.

MEDICATIONS/NUTRIENTS LINKED TO DECREASED THYROID FUNCTION

Sometimes medications or nutrients are associated with a decrease of thyroid function. They may lower absorption of thyroid hormone or elevate the excretion of thyroid hormone. The following are some of the supplements that may alter thyroid function:

- Aluminum hydroxide
- Bile acid sequestrants
- Calcium
- Ferrous sulfate
- Lactose
- Sucralfate

The following are some of the medications that may also alter thyroid function:

- Amiodarone
- Cimetidine
- Clomiphene
- Haloperidol

- Lithium (blocks iodine transport)
- Metoclopramide
- Oral contraceptives

In addition, the following is a partial list of medications that increase the clearance of thyroid hormone so that it leaves the body sooner.

- Carbamezapine
- Phenobarbitol
- Phenytoin
- Rifampin

- Ritonavir
- Sertraline
- Tamoxifen used for more than one year

THYROID HORMONE REPLACEMENT

When you consider thyroid hormone replacement it is important to look at how thyroid hormone is metabolized in the body. The body requires about 50 mg per year of iodine. About 70 percent of the T4 secreted daily is deiodinated to yield T3 and reverse T3 in equal parts. Eighty percent of circulating T3 comes from the peripheral monodeiodination of T4 at the thyrosol ring which occurs in the liver, kidney, and other tissues. Circulating reverse T3 is made the same way. Thyroid hormone is also metabolized in other pathways. It can be conjugated with glucuronate or sulfate and then excreted in the bile or it can be decarboxylated. Twenty percent to 40 percent of T4 is subsequently eliminated in the stool.

Studies have shown that most people do better, if they need thyroid replacement, to have both T3 and T4 replaced. One study of 89 patients with hypothyroidism that were treated with T4 alone previously was compared to a group of people with low thyroid function that were not treated. The symptoms of the patients already on T4 were not any different from the people who were untreated. Their symptoms improved after being treated with desiccated thyroid, which is both T3 and T4. In fact, intracellular thyroid hormone receptors have a high affinity for T3. Ninety percent of the thyroid hormone molecules that bind with the receptors are T3 and 10 percent are T4. Other studies have verified that most individuals have fewer symptoms if they are prescribed both T3 and T4. In another study the lab results were not better, but the patients felt better if they took both T3 and T4.

Prescriptions for Thyroid Replacement

There are different ways to take thyroid hormone replacement. They are all a prescription. You can take T4 alone, take T3 alone, or take both T4 and T3 which is commonly prescribed as desiccated thyroid, which is porcine (from a pig). If you have Hashimoto's thyroiditis, some studies in the medical literature suggest that porcine thyroid replacement may not be the best form to take. This problem can be solved by your doctor prescribing non-porcine thyroid hormone, which is compounded.

Common Desiccated Thyroid Hormones

The following are common desiccated thyroid hormones that are available in North America through a prescription. Most of them are close to four parts T4 to one part T3.

- Armour thyroid (porcine) (ratio: T4 4 to T3 1)

- Euthroid (ratio: T4 4 to T3 1)

- Liotrix (ratio: T4 4 to T3 1)

- S-P-T (pork thyroid suspended in soybean oil)

- Thyroid Strong (ratio: T4 3.1 to T3 1)

- Thyroid USP (ratio: T4 4.2 to T3 1) It may contain lactose sucrose, dextrose or starch—commonly more than 99 percent of the contents are not thyroid hormone

- Thyrolar (ratio: T4 to T3 1)

- Thyrar (bovine)

Common Prescription T4

Listed below are the most common prescription T4 available in North America. All are immediate release and may contain lactose, which can interfere with thyroid hormone absorption. Absorption can vary from 48 to 80 percent.

- Eltroxin

- Levothyroid

- Levoxyl

- Synthroid

Common T3 Medications

The most common T3 medications available in North America all of which are immediate release include:

- Cytomel

- Liothyronine sodium (generic)

- Triostat (injectable)

Compound Thyroid Medication

Compounded thyroid medication is made by a compounding pharmacy that is specially trained to make compounded medications. The advantage to having your thyroid hormone compounded is that you then can have the ratio of your T4 and T3 to be any ratio that you want it to be. Four to one may not be the best ratio for you. In other words, compounded prescription thyroid medication is customized to your own needs. It is personalized. One size does not fit all patients. Also you are getting no fillers and the physician, when they write your prescription for compounded thyroid hormone, can also add selenium, chromium, zinc, iodine, or other nutrients if needed. Recent studies have shown that it is now time for personalized thyroid replacement to be prescribed for patients.

It is paramount that when you are started on thyroid medication that you have your thyroid levels re-measured in six weeks. Once you have an optimal dosage schedule, then you thyroid level should be re-measured every six months since there are things that can change your dose of thyroid medication, such as weight gain or weight loss. The amount of stress that you have also affects your thyroid dosage.

THYROID HORMONE AND THE IMMUNE SYSTEM

As you have just seen, the thyroid hormone regulates most everything that goes on in the body, which also includes the immune system. In fact, thyroid hormones have an extensive effect on the immune system. Growing evidence compiled over recent decades has revealed a two-way crosstalk between thyroid hormones and the immune system. This interplay has been demonstrated for several pathophysiological conditions of thyroid functioning and the innate and adaptive immunity.

Many situations primarily affecting the action of thyroid hormones have an impact on the characteristics and/or functions of immune cells and are translated to host defense status and related disorders. In turn, immune-related disorders lead to the most frequent thyroid dysfunctions, which have an autoimmune origin where the body's immune system attack's itself by mistake. The connection between these systems is complex and not well-understood. This section of the chapter reviews the current evidence supporting the contribution of thyroid hormone to the modulation of innate immunity at the cellular level.

As discussed in Part 1 of this book, the immune system includes cells that protect the organism from foreign antigens, such as microbes, cancer cells, toxins, and damage signals. It is simplistically referred to as innate and adaptive immunity. The former offers immediate protection against intruders, with specific cells being able to fight a wide range of pathogens, with the latter being specific and antigen dependent. Additionally, adaptive immunity is orchestrated and directed by its innate counterpart. The immune effects of T3 and T4 on the body occur in the innate immune cell subsets: neutrophils, natural killer (NK) cells, macrophages, and dendritic cells (DC).

Neutrophils

Neutrophils are the first line of defense against bacteria and fungi. They also help to combat parasites and viruses. They travel from the blood to the inflammatory site where they engage and kill microorganisms and clear infections. This is acomplished through chemotaxis, phagocytosis, and cytokine synthesis, and the release of reactive oxygen species (ROS) and granular proteins, such as myeloperoxidase (MPO). Thyroid hormone metabolism plays an important role in neutrophil function during infection. Likewise, type 3 deiodinase plays a role in the bacterial killing capacity of neutrophils. Recent results have also demonstrated that intracellular thyroid hormone levels are regulated by type 3 deiodinase, playing a key role in neutrophil function.

Natural Killer Cells

Natural killer cells (NK cells) mediate cytolytic activities against tumor and virus-infected targets. In addition, NK cells also possess traits of adaptive immunity and can acquire functional qualities associated with immunological memory. T3 increases NK cell activity and increases IFN-y (type II interferon) response on the NK cell activity, which is critical for innate and adaptive immunity.

Macrophages

The endocrine system plays a part in regulating macrophage maturation. Macrophages are uniquely positioned in all tissues of the body and can recognize and remove pathogens, toxins, cellular debris, and apoptotic cells. Tissue-resident macrophages in adulthood rely on replenishment by bone marrow-derived blood monocytes, with circulating monocytes being recruited to tissues by specific chemical stimuli. Among other names, tissue-resident macrophages are referred to as "microglia" in the central nervous system and

"Kupffer cells" in the liver. Depending on the signal and the dose, a second stimulation can result in tolerance or trained immunity.

As discussed in Chapter 1, in response to stimuli, differentiated macrophages polarize to classically activated M1 or alternatively activated M2 (anti-inflammatory) macrophages. M1 (pro-inflammatory) macrophages engulf and destroy microbes, eliminate tumor cells, and present antigens to T cells through ROS (reactive oxygen species) production, thus promoting T helper (Th) 1 responses and M2 macrophages. These regulatory cells are involved in tissue repair, promote tumor growth, and exert anti-parasitic effects.

Studies have shown the inflammatory response exerted by macrophages became stimulated when a person was hypothyroid. Switching from M1 to the M2 phenotype protects the organism from excessive inflammation. Whereas switching from M2 to M1 prevents allergic and asthmatic Th2 reactions, decreases the bactericidal properties of macrophages and favors the resolution of inflammation. The inhibition of IL-6 (interleuken-6) signaling induced by T3 has potent regulatory functions during infection and inflammation.

Dendritic Cells

Dendritic cells (DC) are the main antigen presenting cells in the connection between innate and adaptive immunity. They integrate signals derived from infection or damage, and present processed antigen to naive T cells—cells that are generated in the thymus waiting to be activated—to tailor the appropriate T cell program. T3 promotes dendritic cell maturation and function which drive pro-inflammatory and cytotoxic adaptive responses. Dendritic cells are involved in the pathogenesis—development of—autoimmune thyroid diseases and also their potential application for the treatment of these pathologies.

CONCLUSION

This chapter provided an overview of the molecular machinery of intracellular thyroid hormone metabolism present in neutrophils, macrophages, and dendritic cells and the role and effects of intracellular thyroid hormone metabolism in these cells. Likewise, as you have seen, circulating thyroid hormone levels have a profound effect on neutrophil, macrophage, and dendritic cell function, This phenomenon suggests that thyroid hormone metabolism plays an important role in the host defense against infection through the modulation of innate immune cell function.

Both under and over production of thyroid hormone can negatively impact the immune system. This chapter discussed the much more common state of low thyroid hormone production, hypothyroidism. Optimal thyroid function requires adequate nutritional intake. It is also related to toxin exposure, other hormonal function, medication usage, stress, and many other factors. In addition, many elements determine optimal thyroid function including accurate measuring techniques. Most individuals that require thyroid replacement benefit from both T3 and T4 to optimize thyroid function and consequently improve overall health. This includes balancing immune function, since thyroid hormones are modulators of the immune response, along with regulators of many of the other functions in your body.

14

Water
Stay Hydrated

The next key to having a health immune system is to drink enough water. Water regulates every function in the body. Without adequate hydration, the body manages less effectively in so many ways. Staying hydrated, not only allows your body to obtain electrolytes and helps your bodily functions to work at optimum levels, but also helps your system naturally remove toxins and other microbes that may result in a number of medical conditions.

Water enables the kidneys to remove toxins; if you don't drink enough water, toxins will accumulate, compromising your immune system. Being hydrated assures that your blood will transfer oxygen to the cells in your body and it allows your cells to take in nutrients. Water aids in the production of lymph, which the body utilizes to circulate white blood cells and nutrients. Nutrition is a key element in maintaining a strong immune system and being hydrated assists in carrying out the digestion of food.

There is no substitute for water. The average adult body is comprised of about 50 to 65 percent water—men composed of more water than women. An adult male's body is 60 to 65 percent water, compared to 50 to 60 percent for an adult female.

CAUSES OF DEHYDRATION

Dehydration occurs when the body is not getting enough water or fluids to replace the water lost. Although our bodies process and lose water at a rate that usually aligns with our metabolism, we can lose fluids at increased rates when we are ill, exercising, sweating heavily, or suffering from other conditions that are caused by the loss of extreme amounts of water.

While there are obvious explanations for why you can end up

dehydrated—a sunny, hot day, exercise, or just not drinking enough—other causes are less clear. There are eight major triggers of dehydration.

- Alcohol use
- Caffeinated beverages
- Exercising and sweating
- Fever
- Increased urination in conditions such as diabetes mellitus and diabetes insipidus
- Injury to the mouth
- Some medications cause an increase in urination such as diuretics (water pills)
- Vomiting or diarrhea

SYMPTOMS OF DEHYDRATION

Becoming dehydrated can be a grave problem for your body. When you use or lose more water than you take in, your body struggles to carry out its normal functions. When you experience thirst, you are already dehydrated. The potential to identify the symptoms associated with dehydration might help you rehydrate sooner. Therefore, it is crucial to recognize the signs and symptoms of not consuming enough water. The following are symptoms and signs of dehydration in an adult:

- Anxiety
- Cognitive changes
- Confusion or feeling dazed
- Dark-colored urine
- Decreased concentration
- Decreased urination
- Dizziness
- Dry mouth
- Fatigue
- Headache
- Increased perception of task difficulty
- Irritability
- Tension

If you have normal kidney function and you do not have congestive heart failure or another disease process that causes you to have fluid overload, the amount of water you should drink is one-half your body weight in ounces every day. If you are exercising, then increase your water intake by another 20 to 40 ounces that day. If you are unsure as to how much water you need to intake every day, ask your healthcare provider.

In a recent Manz study (*see* reference section) individuals that drank less water had an increased risk in the development and progression of metabolic syndrome, diabetes, obesity, chronic kidney disease, high blood pressure, and heart disease. In addition, maintaining good hydration status has been shown to positively affect constipation and decrease the risk of developing kidney stones. Adequate hydration also has a positive role in preventing urinary tract infections, gallstones, mitral valve prolapse, and glaucoma. Moreover, in individuals with asthma it is important to intake enough water.

Drinking more water also helps promote weight loss since it makes you feel full, decreases fluid retention, and aids in burning stored fat. One of my favorite reasons to drink more water is that it helps flush toxins out of your system. Furthermore, intaking additional water helps to hydrate your skin to aid in avoiding wrinkling and encouraging the smoothness and softness of the skin. Lastly, having adequate hydration energizes you and is a great therapy for fatigue.

GETTING WATER FROM YOUR FOODS

By the process of metabolism, you are able to obtain some of the water that is essential through the foods you eat, such as fruits and vegetables. Apart from generally getting about 20 percent of your water each day from food, you also obtain nutrients as well.

If you think that drinking water is boring, then add an orange, lemon, lime, or other fruit to enhance the flavor. However, you can obtain some of the water you need by eating foods with a high water content, such as apples, cherry tomatoes, carrots, and cantaloupe. If you are traveling, minimize your intake of caffeine, sugar, and alcohol in order to stay hydrated.

Even though there is no substitute for water, you can eat your way into hydration. Dr. Dana Cohen in her book, *Quench: Beat Fatigue, Drop Weight, and Heal Your Body Through the Science of Optimum Hydration*, she discusses both veggies and fruits that help hydrate the body in order of water content.

Top 12 Hydrating Veggies

- Cucumbers
- Romaine lettuce
- Celery
- Radishes
- Zucchini
- Tomatoes
- Peppers
- Cauliflower
- Spinach
- Broccoli
- Carrots
- Sprouts

Top 12 Hydrating Fruits

- Apples
- Blueberries
- Cantaloupe
- Grapefruit
- Grapes
- Kiwi

- Pears
- Pineapple

- Raspberries
- Starfruit

- Strawberries
- Watermelon

Foods and drinks to limit, which can dehydrate the body, include the following: alcohol, sugar, and a large portion of grains, starches, meats, cheeses, coffee, and teas. If you partake of these, then compensate with addition water intake. Moderation is the key to health!

CONCLUSION

Staying well hydrated helps to enhance your immune system. As outlined in this chapter, being adequately hydrated promotes better health, reduces fatigue, aids in digestion, oxygenates the blood, flushes toxins out, as well as having a therapeutic effect for many chronic disorders. It allows your body to better defend itself against microbes and to recover more quickly. For an overall well-being, it is important to appropriately hydrate.

PART 3

Herbal and Nutritional Therapies for Immune Building

Part 3 of this book will help facilitate your understanding of ways to build your immune system along with examining nutritional and herbal therapies to help balance your immune system so it functions optimally. This section of the book focuses on nutritional and herbal therapies that aid in immune building.

Natural remedies made from herbs help us take control of our day-to-day well-being and boost the immune system. Herbal therapies include echinacea, glycyrrhizin, elderberry, astragalus, ginseng, oregano, and garlic. Olive leaf extract and cordyceps are also beneficial.

Nutritional therapies, such as zinc, selenium, vitamin D, vitamin A, chromium, and manganese, have been shown to be crucial for the growth and function of immune cells. In addition, other nutritional remedies are available to furthermore build the immune system, such as transfer factor, beta glucans, glutathione, sulforaphane, alpha lipoic acid, modified citrus pectin, and colostrum. Amino acids, such as carnosine, carnitine, arginine, and glutamine, have also been shown to be effective.

Lastly, herbal and nutritional therapies that are centered around building your immunity and decreasing inflammation, such as curcumin, EGCG, fish oil, ginger, pycnogenol, resveratrol, glycyrrhizin, pomegranate, n-acetyl cysteine (NAC), and white willow bark, will be discussed in this part of the book.

HERBAL THERAPIES

The healing properties of herbs are thought to be largely due to their *phyto-nutrients*—chemical compounds found only in plants that develop to protect the plant, but also offer benefits to human beings. In fact, more than 40 percent of the medications used today have been based on phytonutrients, and it is estimated that nearly 80 percent of the world's population uses herbs for some aspect of primary healthcare, such as boosting your immune system.

Regardless of whether you choose pharmaceutical grade herbal supplements or whole herbs, you must utilize them correctly and appropriately. Because herbs are natural, they are often considered safer than prescription drugs. But herbs contain potent substances that can potentially have harmful effects—especially when taken without consideration for proper guidelines and precautions, or when taken with certain medications. Always read all directions before taking an herbal supplement. You should also consult your doctor before starting any supplement regimen—particularly if you have kidney or liver disease or are pregnant or nursing. Your pharmacist is another good source of information about herb and drug interactions.

A supplement's potency is very important, since a low potency usually means that the product will provide you with little or no results. Its potency refers to its concentration of active ingredients and in order for a supplement to be potent it must be absorbed by your body. To test how well it can be absorbed, drop an herbal supplement into a glass of water and watch what happens. The herbs should dissolve. An herb that doesn't dissolve will probably not have consistent potency since it will not be well absorbed. Likewise, your GI tract (gut) must function optimally in order for it to be well absorbed.

There are a variety of different ways to utilize medicinal herbs. Your options include compresses, decoctions (an herbal solution made by cooking hard and woody parts of a plant) and infusions (brew herb, steep, and drink or use to make compresses), drinking teas, poultice (a paste made of ground herbs and oil or warm water that is applied directly to the skin), or tablets and capsules.

ASTRAGALUS

Astragalus (*Astragalus membranaceus*) belongs to the pea family. The astragalus root contains an isoflavone that can enhance metabolism and digestion, as well as treat related problems. Astragalus also contains triterpenoid saponins, substances that are believed to lower cholesterol levels and have antioxidant effects. Furthermore, this herb contains polysaccharides that strengthen the immune system.

■ Functions of Astragalus in Your Body

- Enhances digestion by strengthening the intestine's movement and muscle tone
- Helps regulate the immune system
- Improves sperm motility
- Increases blood flow
- Is an antioxidant
- Lowers blood pressure
- Lowers blood sugar
- Lowers cholesterol
- Protects the liver
- Protects the nerves

■ Conditions That Can Benefit from Astragalus

- Allergies
- Angina
- Asthma
- Cancer (as adjunct to chemotherapy and to decrease side effects)
- Cerebral ischemia (insufficient blood flow to the brain)
- Chronic fatigue syndrome
- Chronic kidney disease
- Cognitive decline
- Congestive heart failure
- Cough, colds, and upper respiratory tract infections
- Diabetes
- Exposure to toxins
- Fibromyalgia
- HIV/AIDS
- Hypercholesterolemia (high cholesterol)
- Hypertension (high blood pressure)
- Kidney dysfunction caused by lithotripsy treatments
- Male infertility
- Stress
- Stroke (post-stroke treatment)
- Viral infection (prevention and treatment)

■ Recommended Dosage

Dose depends on health status, age, renal function, and weight. The following are common doses:

- 250 to 500 milligrams of standardized extract three to four times daily.

- 2 to 4 milliliters 1:1 fluid extract three times daily.

■ Side Effects and Contraindications

Do not take astragalus after an organ transplant or if you have an allergy to gum tragacanth. Astragalus may interact with medications that affect the immune system, such as drugs taken by organ transplant recipients and some cancer patients. It can also interact with steroids and lithium. Speak to your healthcare provider or pharmacist to learn if astragalus might interact with any of the drugs you're taking.

Although astragalus is considered safe for most adults, commonly reported side effects include gastrointestinal issues such as diarrhea.

CORDYCEPS

Cordyceps (*Cordyceps sinsensis* and *Cordyceps militaris*) is a mushroom that has long been used, particularly in traditional Chinese medicine. The main constituent of the extract derived from this fungus is cordycepin (3'deoxy-adenosine). Furthermore, cordyceps contains various types of essential amino acids, vitamins B1, B2, B12 and K, carbohydrates, such as monosaccharide and oligosaccharides, and various polysaccharides, proteins, sterols, nucleosides, and other trace elements.

■ Functions of Cordyceps in Your Body

- Anti-bacterial
- Anti-cancer
- Anti-inflammatory
- Antioxidant
- Helps regulate heart rhythm
- Immunomodulatory (helps to balance the immune system)
- Improves kidney function
- Improves lung capacity
- Increases cardiac output
- Increases energy levels
- Insecticidal
- Interferes in mTOR signal transduction (important in regulating the cell cycle)

- Interferes with purine biosynthesis

- Lowers blood sugar

- Lowers cholesterol

- Lowers fibrinogen (a clotting factor)

- Neuroprotective

- Provokes RNA chain termination

Conditions That Can Benefit from Cordyceps

- Athletic performance

- Cardiac arrhythmias

- Chronic kidney disease

- Cirrhosis

- Congestive heart failure

- Coughs, bronchitis, asthma

- Currently being studied as a possible anti-cancer agent

- Hepatitis B

- Immune building

- Infection

- Sexual enhancement

Recommended Daily Dosage

Dosage depends on concentration of the active ingredient. Common dose is: 500 mg to 1,500 mg a day in divided doses. Some athletes take 3 grams a day.

Side Effects and Contraindications

- Do not take if you are allergic to molds.

- Do not use if you have an autoimmune disease.

- Safety has not been determined in pregnant women or women that are breast-feeding. Therefore, do not use if you are pregnant or breast feeding.

- Taking cordyceps might increase the risk of bleeding in individuals with bleeding disorders or people on medications that change bleeding time. Use with caution.

- Taking cordyceps might make the drug prednisolone less effective.

- There has been couple of reports on lead poisoning in patients taking cordyceps. Make sure you take a pharmaceutical grade product.

- Use cordyceps with caution if you are taking anti-viral or diabetic medications since this mushroom can affect the dosage of these drugs.

- Using cordyceps might increase the risk of bleeding during surgery. Therefore, discontinue taking cordyceps 2 weeks before surgery.

ECHINACEA

The North American plant echinacea was long used as traditional medicine by Native Americans of the Great Plains. Now, scientific research shows that this herb is notable in its ability to enhance the immune system and help ward off colds and resist infections. Echinacea is also used in topical preparations that are applied to the skin. There are three types of echinacea that are commonly used for medicinal purposes: *angustifolia*, *pallida*, and *purpurea*.

▓ Functions of Echinacea in Your Body

- Boosts immune system
- Fights colds and flu
- Helps heal damaged skin
- Is an anti-inflammatory
- Protects skin from sun damage

▓ Conditions That Can Benefit from Echinacea

- Acne
- Allergies
- Bronchial asthma
- Burns
- Cancer
- Candidiasis
- Colic
- Common colds (prevention and treatment)
- Compromised immune system
- Eczema
- Flu
- Halitosis
- Herpes
- Radiation-induced leukopenia
- Sore throat
- Upper respiratory infections
- Urinary tract infections
- Wounds

▓ Recommended Daily Dosage

- When taken for general well-being, take 250 to 500 milligrams orally every day for no longer than eight weeks in a row.
- When taken to fight a cold for which the symptoms have already begun, take 1 to 2 grams orally every day. Start as soon as possible after noticing the symptoms. Continue treatment for three weeks.
- When used to heal a burn or wound, apply topically to injured area daily. If improvement is not seen after one week, discontinue therapy.

■ Side Effects and Contraindications

• Some people experience dizziness or nausea when taking echinacea.

• Anaphylaxis, asthma exacerbation, and angio-edema have been reported in rare cases.

• Individuals should not use this herb if they are allergic to sunflowers, daisies, marigolds, chrysanthemums, or dandelions.

• Use echinacea with caution if you have an autoimmune disease.

• No significant herb-drug interactions with echinacea have been reported. Based on in vitro studies, echinacea may be a mild inhibitor of the cytochrome P450 3A4 enzyme complex system. Therefore, use echinacea with caution if you are taking a medication that clears through the liver.

ELDERBERRY

Black elderberry (*Sambucus nigra*) has been used for many years to prevent and treat influenza. The berries are dark violet-black drupes which grow in clusters and owe their color to the anthocyanins; a group of phenolic compounds which are abundant in elderberries and considered the active constituents of the fruits. In addition, elderberries contain a variety of nutrients ranging from vitamins (A, B1, B2, B6, B9, C and E), trace elements such as zinc, copper, iron and minerals such as calcium and magnesium. Furthermore, elderberry contains carotenoids, phytosterols, and polyphenols. These additional constituents give elderberry unique functions.

■ Functions of Elderberry in Your Body

• Activates the immune system by increasing the production of inflammatory cytokines (IL-1 beta, TNF-alpha, IL-6, IL-8)

• Antibacterial (against both gram-positive Strep and Branhamella in cultures)

• Antidepressant

• Antidiabetic

• Anti-inflammatory

• Antioxidant

• Anti-viral

• Immune modulating

• Immuno-protective or immunostimulatory

■ Conditions That Can Benefit from Elderberry

• Bacterial infections

• Cancer

- Constipation

- Herpes simplex

- Immune builder

- Prevention and treatment of influenza (reduces symptoms and duration)

- Sinusitis

- Upper respiratory infection

◼ Recommended Daily Dosage

The dose selection is based on dosages used by popular elderberry products, which range from 650 mg to 1500 mg per day. The most common dose is to take two capsules per day (600 mg) during the priming phase (before travel, –10 until –2 days) and three capsules per day (900 mg) while travelling and overseas (–1 until +4 days).

◼ Side Effects and Contraindications

- Elderberry fruit extract is safe when taken by mouth for up to three months.

- There is not enough information to know if elderberry is safe to use when pregnant or breast-feeding. Therefore, do not use if you are pregnant or breast feeding.

- Use with caution if you have an autoimmune disease.

- Elderberry can increase the immune system. Taking elderberry along with some medications that decrease the immune system might decrease the effectiveness of these medications:

  - Azathioprine
  - Basiliximab
  - Cyclosporine
  - Daclizumab
  - Muromonab-CD3

  - Mycophenolate
  - Sirolimus
  - Steroids
  - Tacrolimus

GARLIC

For thousands of years, garlic (*Allium sativum*) has been known to offer a variety of medicinal benefits. This pungent bulb is packed with nutrients, including amino acids, vitamins, trace minerals, flavonoids, enzymes, and two hundred additional compounds. Most of garlic's health benefits, though, are the result of its sulfur compounds, the most famous of which is allicin, an antibacterial that is produced when the garlic is crushed or chopped. Because allicin is most effective immediately after its formation, garlic should be eaten soon after it is prepared. Garlic supplements containing allicin are also available.

■ Functions of Garlic in Your Body

- Balances blood sugar levels
- Boosts your immune system by increasing natural killer cell activity
- Decreases LDL (bad) cholesterol and increases HDL (good) cholesterol
- Decreases plasma viscosity
- Increases cellular glutathione synthesis
- Increases nitric oxide, which increases blood flow
- Is a natural blood thinner
- Is a powerful anti-inflammatory
- Is an antioxidant
- Lowers blood pressure
- Lowers homocysteine, decreasing the risk of heart disease, osteoporosis, depression, and memory loss
- Lowers triglyceride levels
- May decrease the risk of prostate cancer

■ Conditions That Can Benefit from Garlic

- Atherosclerosis
- Cancer (colon, esophageal, and stomach)
- Common cold (prevention)
- Heart disease
- Hypercholesterolemia (high cholesterol)
- Hyperhomocysteinemia (high homocysteine)
- Hypertension (high blood pressure)
- Infection

■ Recommended Dosage

10 milligrams allicin or a total allicin potential of 4,000 micrograms (equal to one clove of garlic).

■ Side Effects and Contraindications

Garlic is a blood thinner. If you are taking a blood-thinning medication or a supplement that is a blood thinner, do not take garlic supplements and do not eat large amounts of garlic. Garlic can also interact with blood pressure medication. Speak to your healthcare provider or pharmacist to learn if any drugs you're taking might make it unwise to take garlic supplements.

Pregnant women should not take large doses of garlic—fresh or in supplement form—since sizeable amounts of garlic can cause uterine contractions.

Possible side effects of garlic ingestion include the following:

- Abdominal pain
- Allergic conjunctivitis, rhinitis, or bronchospasms
- Bad breath
- Bloating
- Diarrhea
- Dizziness
- Gas
- Headache
- Heartburn
- Nausea/vomiting
- Profuse sweating

GINSENG

Ginseng is a family of herbs well known for its strong medicinal benefits. There are two popular types of this plant: American ginseng and Asian ginseng, which is often called Korean or Chinese ginseng. The two varieties have many similar medicinal effects, and both contain ginsenosides, the active ingredients in ginseng. Both varieties are also adaptogens, which means that they help you adapt to stress by exerting a normalizing effect on your body's processes. This is why the herb can, for instance, correct both low and high levels of cortisol. Yet the two ginseng varieties are sufficiently different in their effects to warrant separate discussions.

Note that Siberian ginseng, or eleuthero (*Eleutherococcus senticosus*), is a different plant and does not have the same active ingredients. (*See* page 210 for a discussion of eleuthero.)

AMERICAN GINSENG

American ginseng (*Panax quinquefolium*), which grows chiefly in North America, is valued for several biological activities, including the management of stress, boosting the immune system, and increasing energy.

■ Functions of American Ginseng in Your Body

- Helps control menopausal symptoms
- Increases energy

- Is an adaptogen that helps the body manage stress
- Is an antioxidant
- Lowers blood sugar levels

- Lowers insulin levels
- May improve memory
- Strengthens the immune system

Conditions That Can Benefit from American Ginseng

- Attention-deficit/hyperactivity disorder (ADHD)
- Cancer-related fatigue
- Cognition problems
- Common cold (prevention)
- Diabetic neuropathy (numbness and tingling of the extremities due to diabetes)

- Heart disease
- Hypercortisolism (high cortisol)
- Hypocortisolism (low cortisol)
- Hypertension (high blood pressure)
- Insulin resistance/diabetes

Recommended Dosage

125 to 500 milligrams. Take ginseng with food so that it doesn't lower your blood sugar levels too dramatically. Do not take this supplement consistently for more than one year.

Side Effects and Contraindications

Do not take ginseng if you are taking warfarin or another blood-thinning medication, as ginseng can decrease the effectiveness of the medication. Also avoid ginseng if you are pregnant or breastfeeding, or if you have a history of breast cancer or other hormone-sensitive conditions.

American ginseng can interact with a wide range of drugs, including blood thinners, MAO inhibitors, diabetes medication, drugs used to treat ADHD, and more. Speak to your healthcare provider or pharmacist to learn if any of the medications you're taking might make it unwise to use American ginseng supplements.

Ginseng can make the effects of caffeine stronger, possibly causing nervousness, sweating, insomnia, or irregular heartbeat. Avoid caffeine or stop taking ginseng if you experience these symptoms.

Common side effects of ginseng include the following:

- Anxiety
- Breast pain

- Diarrhea
- Euphoria

- Headache
- Hypertension (high blood pressure)
- Insomnia

- Nosebleed
- Restlessness
- Vaginal bleeding
- Vomiting

ASIAN GINSENG

Asian ginseng (*Panax ginseng*), also called Chinese ginseng and Korean ginseng, is available in two forms: red and white. These forms are derived from the same species but are different because of the way the plant is processed. Both are dried, but red ginseng is steamed after drying. Although both forms are common, red ginseng is preferred for medicinal purposes because the processing actually raises the level of certain ginsenosides in the plant.

■ Functions of Asian Ginseng in Your Body

- Aids in lowering cholesterol and triglycerides
- Decreases bloating and fullness
- Decreases depression
- Enhances heart function
- Enhances liver function
- Helps increase physical endurance
- Helps relieve anxiety
- Helps relieve insomnia and restlessness

- Improves glucose control
- Improves mood
- Increases energy
- Increases mental abilities
- Is an adaptogen that helps the body manage stress
- Is an antioxidant
- May improve memory
- Strengthens the immune system
- Supports adrenal function

■ Conditions That Can Benefit from Asian Ginseng

- Acne
- AIDS
- Cancer (prevention and decrease of chemotherapy side effects)
- Chronic fatigue syndrome

- Chronic obstructive pulmonary disease (COPD)
- Depression
- Erectile dysfunction
- Hair loss

- Hearing loss due to medications such as cisplatin and aminoglycosides (prevention)

- Hypercholesterolemia (high cholesterol)

- Hypercortisolism (high cortisol level)

- Hypertriglyceridemia (high triglycerides)

- Hypocortisolism (low cortisol level)

- Insulin resistance/diabetes

- Memory loss (prevention)

- Stomach ulcers (prevention)

- Wounds

■ Recommended Dosage

125 to 500 milligrams. Take ginseng with food so that it doesn't lower your blood sugar levels too dramatically. Do not take this supplement consistently for more than one year.

■ Side Effects and Contraindications

Do not take Asian ginseng if you have bipolar disorder, because this supplement can increase the risk of mania. Also avoid ginseng if you are pregnant or breastfeeding, or if you have a history of breast cancer or other hormone-sensitive conditions.

Asian ginseng can interact with a wide range of drugs, including blood thinners, MAO inhibitors, ACE inhibitors, drugs used after organ transplants, drugs used to treat ADHD, and more. Speak to your healthcare provider or pharmacist to learn if any medications you're taking might make it unwise to use ginseng supplements.

Asian ginseng may make the effects of caffeine stronger, possibly causing nervousness, sweating, insomnia, or irregular heartbeat. Avoid caffeine or stop taking ginseng if you experience these symptoms.

Common side effects of ginseng include the following:

- Breast pain

- Diarrhea

- Euphoria

- Headache

- Hypertension (high blood pressure)

- Nosebleed

- Vaginal bleeding

- Vomiting

GOLDENSEAL

One of the top-selling herbs in the United States, goldenseal (*Hydrastis canadensis*) is native to North America, and its roots have a range of medicinal uses. The benefits of goldenseal are derived from the plant's many constituents, which include amino acids; alkaloids, such as berberine, hydrastine, and canalidine, and more. Generally, the alkaloid content is used as a marker for standardization and quality control.

■ Functions of Goldenseal in Your Body

- Boosts immune function
- Cleans and treats sore or inflamed gums and canker sores
- Has potent cancer cell-killing activity
- Helps to detoxify the body
- Improves digestive issues through antimicrobial activity
- Is an anti-inflammatory
- Kills pathogens in the body, including bacterium, fungus, and virus
- Lowers blood glucose levels
- Relieves congestion
- Stimulates antibodies

■ Conditions That Can Benefit from Goldenseal

- Alcohol-related liver disease
- Allergies
- Alzheimer's disease (decreases beta-amyloid peptides)
- Arthritis
- Atherosclerosis
- Bladder infection
- Canker sores, recurrent
- Colds
- Congestive heart failure
- Constipation
- Depression
- Diarrhea
- Eczema
- Hypercholesterolemia (high cholesterol)
- Indigestion
- Inflammation
- Insulin resistance/diabetes
- Irregular heartbeat (arrhythmia)
- Polycystic ovary syndrome (PCOS)
- Psoriasis
- Radiation-induced intestinal symptoms (prevention)

- Radiation-induced lung injury (prevention)
- Sore throat

- Stomach problems
- Vaginitis/yeast infections
- Wounds

Recommended Dosage

Goldenseal can be taken orally—as a capsule, tea, or liquid extract—or used as a topical cream. Orally, take 250 to 500 milligrams two to three times a day. Be sure to take B-complex vitamin supplements during treatment, and do not take goldenseal for longer than two weeks. Then, allow a break of at least two weeks before using goldenseal again. If using a topical cream, follow the manufacturer's directions.

Side Effects and Contraindications

Do not take goldenseal if you are pregnant or nursing, if you have kidney or liver disease, or if you have high blood pressure.

Goldenseal can interact with a wide range of drugs, including blood thinners, tetracycline antibiotics, medication used after organ transplants, digoxin, and more. Speak to your healthcare provider or pharmacist to learn if any medications you're taking might make it unwise to use goldenseal.

Although allergic reactions to goldenseal are rare, they have been occasionally reported. Stop taking this supplement and seek medical attention if you experience any of the following symptoms:

- Breathing difficulty
- Closing of the throat

- Hives
- Swelling of the lips, tongue, or face

Large doses of goldenseal can be toxic and can cause cardiac damage, paralysis, respiratory failure, seizures, and even death. If you experience any of the following side effects, stop taking goldenseal and see your doctor.

- Anxiety
- Diarrhea
- Hypotension (low blood pressure)

- Nausea/vomiting
- Seizures
- Shortness of breath

GLYCYRRHIZIN

Licorice (*Glycyrrhiza glabra* or *Glycyrrhiza uralensis*) is an herb grown in the Mediterranean and other parts of the world. The main phytochemicals of licorice include glycyrrhizin, liquiritigenin, coumarins, stilbenoids, fatty acids, phenols, and sterols. Glycyrrhizin is metabolized by the intestinal flora into its pharmacologically active form, glycyrrhetinic acid. There are two types of licorice available. Deglycyrrhizinated licorice (DGL) is used to treat stomach ailments. Glycyrrhizia-containing licorice is used to treat adrenal dysfunction and other medical conditions. Recent studies have shown it has a strong anti-viral effect. This section will discuss only the glycyrrhiza-containing form.

▓ Functions of Glycyrrhizin in Your Body

- Anti-allergic
- Antibacterial
- Anticoagulation effect (inhibits thrombin)
- Antidepressant (functions as a serotonin reuptake inhibitor—SSRI)
- Antifungal
- Anti-inflammatory (down regulates proinflammatory cytokines)
- Antioxidant
- Anti-parasitic
- Antispasmodic
- Antiplatelet effect (prevents blood clots)
- Antitussive
- Anti-ulcer
- Antiviral
- Diminishes monocyte migration towards supernatants of H5N1-infected A549 cells
- Induces interferon gamma in T cells
- Inhibits H5N1-induced expression of the pro-inflammatory molecules CXCL10, interleukin 6, CCL2, and CCL5
- Inhibits phosphorylating enzymes in vesicular stomatitis virus infection
- Interferes with H5N1 replication
- Reduces activation of NFkB, JNK, and p38, redox-sensitive signaling events needed for influenza A virus replication
- Reduces membrane fluidity leading to inhibition of fusion of the viral membrane of HIV-1 with the cell
- Reduces transport to the membrane and sialylation (introduction of one or more silyl groups into a molecule) of hepatitis B virus surface antigen
- Reduces viral latency

- Binds angiotensin-converting enzyme II (ACE 2) which lowers blood pressure
- Decreases the over production of airway exudates
- Expectorant
- Fights cancer
- Helps with sedation
- Immunomodulatory (positive affect on cytokine storm)
- Inhibits the accumulation of intracellular reactive oxygen species (ROS)
- Liver protective
- Mineralocorticoid effect
- Influences steroid metabolism to maintain blood pressure and volume and to regulate glucose/glycogen balance
- Lowers blood sugar
- Lowers cholesterol

- Maintains cognition
- Neuroprotective
- Phytoestrogen (estrogen-like effect)
- Contains isoflavones including licochalcone A which has estrogenic activity
- Liquiritigenin and isoliquirtigenin both have estrogenic activity
- Stimulates aromatase activity which promotes estrogen synthesis
- Protects against cisplatin-induced nephrotoxicity and genotoxicity
- Promotes weight loss
- Inhibits adipogenesis (formation of fatty tissue) through inhibition of C/EBP-alpha and PPAR-alpha
- Stimulatory effect on the adrenal gland (increase cortisol levels)

▓ Conditions That Can Benefit from Glycyrrhizin

- Allergies
- Aphthous ulcers
- Bronchitis
- Cancer
- Carpel tunnel syndrome
- Chronic fatigue syndrome (CFS)
- Depression
- Eczema (atopic dermatitis)
- Epstein-Barr virus

- Hair product (decreases oiliness in the hair)
- Hepatitis B and C
- HIV infection
- Hyperprolactinemia
- Hypocortisolism (low cortisol level)
- May be effective against coronavirus-2 (SARS-CoV-2). It is currently being studied due to its positive effect on cytokine storm.

- Mediterranean fever (Licorice is taken in combination with Siberian ginseng, and Schizandra to treat familial Mediterranean fever.)

- Menopausal symptoms

- Metabolic syndrome

- Oral lichen planus

- Polycystic ovary disease (PCOS) (Licorice is also taken by mouth in combination with peony to increase fertility in patient with PCOS.)

- Preventing diabetes complications

- Psoriasis (improves skin pealing)

- Respiratory tract infections

- Seasonal influenza

- Weight loss

▪ Recommended Daily Dosage

Oral dosage

- Dose will depend on form that licorice is given and clinical condition it is being used for.

- Licorice can be used as a tablet, fluid extract, or tea.

- Licorice extracts should contain more than 30 mg/mL.

Transdermal dosage

- For eczema (atopic dermatitis): gel products containing 1 percent or 2 percent licorice root extract applied three times a day for two weeks

▪ Side Effects and Contraindications

- Contact dermatitis may occur with topic use.

- Discontinue licorice two weeks before surgery and do not restart until two weeks after surgery.

- Do not take if you have high blood pressure. If you develop high blood pressure while taking it, then discontinue.

- Do not use if you have heart disease or an irregular heart rhythm.

- Do not use if you have hypertonia (excessively high muscle tone which causes trembling, involuntary motions, stiffness, and lack of flexibility). Glycyrrhizin may make this condition worse.

- Do not use if you have kidney disease.

- Do not use if you have low potassium levels.

- Do not use in pregnancy.
- Glycyrrhizin may cause water and sodium retention.
- Glycyrrhizin when applied to the skin may cause a rash.
- It may cause:
  - Fatigue
  - Headaches
  - Irregular menstrual cycles due to its estrogenic effect
  - Low potassium levels
- It may decrease sexual interest in men since it can lower testosterone.
- It may exacerbate erectile dysfunction.
- Since licorice has estrogenic effects do not use if you have breast, ovarian, or uterine cancer.
- Use with caution if you have endometriosis or fibroids due to its estrogenic effect.
- Other side effects that may occur include the following:
  - Carpel tunnel syndrome (rarely)
  - Rhabdomyolysis
  - Thrombocytopenia (low platelet count)
  - Increased sodium retention
  - Visual disturbance (with high dose use)
- There are several possible drug interactions that may occur with glycyr-rhizin: both positive and negative effects:
  - Digoxin (interactions are mediated by organic anion-transporting polypeptide 1B1/1B3 in the liver)
  - Diuretics (water pills) that reduce potassium in the body
  - Do not use licorice with cyclosporine since it may reduce the bioavailability of this drug.
  - Ethacrynic acid due to its potassium lowering effects
  - Glycyrrhizin has a positive effect on clotrimazole, an antifungal medication, used to treat Candida albicans.
  - Glycyrrhizin may affect any medication broken down by the liver by increasing or decreasing its breakdown.
  - Glycyrrhizin may decrease the effectiveness of any drug used for hypertension.

- Glycyrrhizin may reduce the effect of potassium supplementation.
- It displays a bio-enhancing effect by significantly increasing the bioactivity of antibiotics such as; tetracycline, ampicillin, rifampicin, and nalidixic acids against gram-positive bacteria (Bacillus subtilis and Mycobacterium smegmatis) and gram negative bacteria (Escherichia coli).
- It enhances the action of H2 antagonists drugs used for reflux.
- It increases the effects of paclitaxel and vinblastine which are medications used for chemotherapy.
- May interfere with oral contraceptives and estrogen replacement
- Use licorice only under a doctor's direction if you are taking methotrexate since it may potentiate the medication's toxicity.
- Warfarin (may increase the breakdown and therefore decrease the effectiveness)

OLIVE LEAF EXTRACT

Extracted from the leaves of the olive tree (*Olea europaea*), olive leaf extract is rich in the plant chemical oleuropein, which is thought to contribute to the anti-inflammatory and antioxidant properties of this medicinal. In fact, the extract contains a number of bioactive components—secoiridoids, flavonoids, and triterpenes being a few—that make it highly valued throughout the world.

Functions of Olive Leaf Extract in Your Body

- Decreases endothelial dysfunction—a pathological state of the endothelium that increases the risk of heart disease
- Decreases the risk of cancer through several mechanisms
- Fights viral and bacterial infections
- Functions as an ACE inhibitor
- Helps prevent tissue-damaging glycation
- Is an anti-inflammatory
- Is an antioxidant
- Lowers blood pressure
- Lowers blood sugar levels by slowing the digestion of starches and increasing the absorption of glucose into the tissues
- Prevents the buildup of uric acid, helping to prevent gout
- Protects the nervous system

■ Conditions That Can Benefit from Olive Leaf Extract

- Cancer prevention
- Gout
- Hypercholesterolemia (high cholesterol)
- Hypertension (high blood pressure)

- Insulin resistance/diabetes
- Osteoarthritis
- Problems with cognitive function
- Rheumatoid arthritis

■ Recommended Dosage

500 milligrams daily. Always take with food to prevent stomach irritation.

■ Side Effects and Contraindications

Since this herb can have blood pressure-lowering and blood glucose-lowering effects, use with caution if you are taking medications to treat these conditions. Speak to your healthcare provider or pharmacist to learn if any drugs you're using might make it wise to avoid olive leaf extract.

Side effects from olive leaf extract use are typically mild and last for only a few days. They may include:

- Diarrhea
- Dizziness

- Heartburn
- Stomach irritation

OREGANO

Oregano (*Origanum vulgare*) leaves and oil contain carvacrol, thymol, eugenol, and rosmarinic acid. This herb has been used for medicinal purposes for thousands of years for respiratory and gastrointestinal disorders and as an antimicrobial.

■ Functions of Oregano in Your Body

- Activates peroxisome proliferator-activated receptors (PPARs)
- Antibiotic
- Antimalarial
- Antioxidant

- Antiviral
- Decreases inflammation
- Increases immune system
- Lowers cholesterol
- Regulates blood sugar

■ Conditions That May Benefit From Oregano

- Aching muscles
- Allergies
- Arthritis
- Bronchitis
- Common cold
- Diabetes
- Diarrhea
- Ear infections
- Fungal infections
- Gingivitis

- Headaches
- Mild depression
- Painful menstrual cramps
- Rheumatoid arthritis
- Sinus infections
- Sinus infections
- Small intestinal bowel overgrowth (SIBO)
- Urinary tract infections

■ Skin Conditions That May Benefit from Diluted Topical Oregano Oil

- Acne
- Athlete's foot
- Dandruff
- Insect bites (can also be used as an insect repellant)
- May promote wound healing

- Psoriasis
- Ringworm
- Rosacea
- Varicose veins
- Warts
- Canker sores

■ Recommended Dosage

The dosage will depend on the usage of oregano as a plant or as an oil.

- Use oregano on salads, steamed or sautéed vegetables, and meat dishes or put dried or fresh oregano in soups, stews, and bone broths. You can also add free oregano leaves to vegetable juice.

- As an oil, put one small drop of oregano essential oil in 8 to 12 ounces of water for sore throats. Make sure you always read the directions on the bottle before use. If using as an essential oil, make sure the oregano oil is always diluted. It may also be combined with other essential oils. In addition, diluted oregano oil can be applied topically for skin conditions. Again, make sure that the oil is diluted no matter what purpose it is being used for, and how it is being used. **Undiluted oregano oil can be lethal.**

■ Side Effects and Contraindications

- Oregano may negatively affect the body's ability to absorb iron, copper, and zinc.

- Avoid oregano for two weeks before surgery, as it can increase the risk of bleeding.

- Do not use for one week after surgery.

- Consult your healthcare provider before starting oregano if you are taking any medication to see if there is a possible herb-drug interaction that may occur.

- Oregano may lower your blood sugar. If you are taking a medication to lower your blood sugar you may need less medication. Therefore, make sure you check your blood sugar on a regular basis especially when you first start this herb.

- If you are using oregano oil, do not swallow or apply directly to the skin. Make sure you dilute essential oils before use.

- If you have an allergy to plants belonging to the Lamiaceae family, which include oregano, basil, lavender, mint, and sage you may have or develop an allergic reaction to oregano.

- Do not use in pregnancy or if you are breast-feeding.

NUTRITIONAL THERAPIES

A deficiency of dietary protein or amino acids has long been known to impair immune function and increase the susceptibility to infectious disease. Recently, the underlying cellular and molecular mechanisms have begun to unfold.

Protein malnutrition reduces concentrations of most amino acids in plasma. Amino acids play an important role in immune responses by regulating: (1) the activation of T lymphocytes, B lymphocytes, natural killer cells, and macrophages; (2) cellular redox state, gene expression and lymphocyte proliferation; and (3) the production of antibodies, cytokines and other cytotoxic substances.

Increasing evidence shows that dietary supplementation of specific amino acids to people with malnutrition and infectious disease enhances the immune status, thereby reducing morbidity and mortality. Arginine, glutamine, and cysteine precursors are the best prototypes. Because of a possible negative impact of imbalance and antagonism among amino acids on nutrient intake and utilization having your amino acid levels measured is suggested before you begin an amino acid therapy program. These nutrients hold great promise in improving the immune system and preventing infectious diseases.

ARGININE

Arginine is an amino acid that can be synthesized in the body from ornithine. Some bodybuilders take arginine supplements because it increases muscle mass while decreasing body fat. In addition, it is also involved in a number of essential bodily functions.

Functions of Arginine in Your Body

- Builds muscle
- Decreases platelet stickiness
- Enhances fat metabolism
- Enhances immune function by increasing natural killer cell activity
- Helps wounds heal
- Important for GI health
- Increase human growth hormone (HGH) production
- Increases circulation
- Increases sperm count
- Inhibits plaque accumulation in the arteries

- Needed for protein production
- Reduces pain from claudication (pain in extremities due to poor circulation)
- Used to produce nitric oxide
- Vital for secretion of glucagon and insulin

Signs and Symptoms of Arginine Deficiency

- Constipation
- Fatty liver
- Hair loss and breakage
- Hepatic cirrhosis
- Poor wound healing
- Skin rash
- Weight gain

Causes of Arginine Deficiency

- Decreased dietary intake in foods that are high in arginine.
- Decreased dietary intake in foods and nutrients that make ornithine.

Conditions That Can Benefit from Arginine

- Anal fissures
- Anemia associated with renal disease
- Body building/improving athletic performance
- Cerebral vascular disease
- Congestive heart failure
- Chronic cyclosporine nephrotoxicity
- Coronary heart disease
- Diabetics
- Improves blood flow to extremities
- May help heal diabetic foot ulcers if used transdermally (on the skin)
- May improve blood sugar control
- Erectile dysfunction
- Fertility (male) (increases sperm count and motility)
- Hyperhomocysteinemia (high homocysteine)
- Hypertension
- Hypertriglyceridemia
- Improves wound healing
- Increases growth hormone production
- Intermittent claudication
- Interstitial cystitis
- Migraine headaches
- Used with ibuprofen
- Malaria
- Post heart transplant

- Using for 6 weeks post-transplant may increase walking distance (consult your doctor before using)

- Polycystic ovarian disease

- Studies have shown that taking n-acetyl cysteine and arginine daily for 6 months can improve menses and reduce insulin resistance.

- Prevention of extreme weight loss in patients with HIV (used with other amino acids)

- Prevention of pressure ulcers in hip-fracture patients

- Raynaud's phenomenon

- Senile dementia

- Sickle cell disease

- Stress

- Early research suggests that taking a combination of lysine and arginine for up to 10 days reduces stress and anxiety.

- Systemic sclerosis

Recommended Daily Dosage

1,000 to 3,000 milligrams daily. There is no standard dose. The amount you may need is based on your body's daily requirements of arginine. If you have heart disease or kidney disease, consult with your doctor to find out the perfect dose for you.

Side Effects and Contraindications

- Arginine can cause an increase in outbreaks of herpes simplex infections: cold sores or genital herpes. The addition of the amino acid lysine to the supplementation program can limit this effect.

- Arginine has unpredictable effects on insulin and cholesterol-lowering agents.

- Arginine may potentiate the effects of isosorbide mononitrate and other nitric oxide donors, such as glyceryl trinitrate and sodium nitroprusside. Therefore, do not use these drugs in conjunction with arginine.

- Discontinue the use of arginine two weeks before surgery since it may have a negative impact on blood pressure.

- Do not use with sildenafil or similar medications.

- Other possible side effects:
  - Abdominal pain
  - Allergies
  - Bitter taste
  - Bloating
  - Blood abnormalities
  - Diarrhea

- Gout
- Hypotension
- Hypotension
- Nausea

- Tightness in chest or throat
- May worsen asthma: therefore, use with caution in patients with asthma

▪ Food Sources

- Asparagus
- Avocados
- Beans
- Broccoli
- Chocolate
- Corn
- Dairy products
- Eggs

- Fish
- Green peas
- Legumes
- Meat
- Nuts
- Oatmeal
- Onion
- Potatoes

- Raisins
- Sesame seeds
- Spinach
- Sunflower seeds
- Swiss chard
- Whey
- Whole grains

CARNITINE

Carnitine is made from lysine and methionine in your liver, kidneys, and brain. Therefore, your being deficient in carnitine implies that you may lack lysine and methionine. Iron, niacin, vitamin B_6, and vitamin C are also necessary to make carnitine. As you age you tend to make less carnitine.

▪ Functions of Carnitine in Your Body

- Can be converted to acetyl choline
- Energizes the heart
- Enhances short- and long-term memory
- Helps convert stored body fat into energy
- Improves mental focus and energy
- Increases oxygen availability and respiratory efficiency

- Lowers LDL cholesterol
- May slow the progression of Alzheimer's disease
- Needed for the transport of long-chain fatty acids into the cells
- Prevents DNA degeneration
- Promotes DNA repair from mutations that occur from free radical production
- Raises HDL cholesterol

- Reduces triglycerides
- Reduces the build-up of acids and metabolic waste

Signs and Symptoms of Carnitine Deficiency

The individual may have no symptoms, or they may be quite severe. They may include the following:

- Decreased or floppy muscle tone
- Edema
- Fatigue
- Irritability
- Muscle weakness
- Shortness of breath

Causes of Carnitine Deficiency

- Deficiency of folic acid
- Deficiency of S-adenosylmethionine (SAMe)
- Deficiency of vitamins B6, B12, and C
- Digestive disease that prevent adequate absorption of nutrients
- Ipecac syrup
- Iron deficiency
- Kidney disease
- Liver disease
- Lysine deficiency
- Malnutrition
- Mitochondrial disease
- Vegetarian diet

Medications

- Avacavir
- Delavirdine
- Didanosine
- Lamivudine
- Nevirapine
- Pivampicillin
- Pyrimethamine
- Stavudine
- Sulfadiazine
- Valproic acid
- Zalcitabine
- Zidovudine

Conditions That Can Benefit from Carnitine

- Alzheimer's disease
- Angina pectoris
- Attention deficit disorder (ADD)
- Brain injuries
- Congestive heart failure
- Depression

- Diabetic neuropathy
- Erectile dysfunction
- High cholesterol levels
- Hyperthyroidism
- Immune enhancement
- Increased triglycerides
- Infertility (increases sperm count and motility)
- Memory enhancement
- Mitral valve prolapse

- Narcolepsy
- Nerve injury
- Parkinson's disease
- Peyronie's disease
- Recovery from heart attack or stroke
- Renal disease
- Senility
- Stroke

Recommended Daily Dosage

500 to 4,000 milligrams daily with normal renal function.

Carnitine comes in three forms:

- Acetyl-L-carnitine: often used in studies for Alzheimer disease and other brain disorders

- Carnitine: the most widely available

- Propionyl-L-carnitine: often used in studies for heart disease and peripheral vascular disease

Avoid D-carnitine supplements. They interfere with the natural form of carnitine and may produce side effects.

Side Effects and Contraindications

Although side effects of carnitine supplementation are rare, they include agitation, headache, increased appetite, nausea, skin rash, dizziness, and vomiting. Some people also experience body odor, which can be prevented by taking riboflavin. If you have kidney or liver disease the dosage of carnitine may need to be reduced or you may not be able to take carnitine as a supplement. In addition, taking carnitine may increase the risk of seizures in individuals with a history of seizure disorder. Carnitine may also increase the risk of bleeding in people taking blood thinning medications. If you have elevated TMAO levels, you may not be able to take carnitine. Therefore, it is always best to check with your healthcare provider before taking this important amino acid.

- Nutrients that increase carnitine effectiveness:
  - Alpha-lipoic acid
  - B vitamins
  - Docosahexaenoic acid (DHA)
  - Eicosapentaenoic acid (EPA)
  - Phosphatidylcholine (PC)
  - Phosphatidylserine (PS)

CHROMIUM

The micronutrient chromium is essential to your health, but your body has a difficult time absorbing it when it is by itself. Combining it with another substance, such as the protein picolinate, allows it to enter the blood stream more easily. Picolinate also increases the absorption of zinc, copper, and iron.

Functions of Chromium in Your Body

- Aids in fat loss
- Burns calories
- Decreases total cholesterol and low-density (bad) cholesterol
- Helps decrease sugar cravings
- Helps hold onto calcium and prevent osteoporosis
- Helps increase the hormone dehydroepiandrosterone (DHEA), which has many roles as a steroid hormone but is also believed to be effective against several diseases
- Helps regulate blood sugar by making insulin work more effectively
- Increases antibodies
- Increases high-density (good) cholesterol
- Increases physical endurance
- Lowers excess cortisol
- Reduces bone loss
- Stimulates muscle development

Symptoms of Chromium Deficiency

- Decreased insulin binding and receptor number, which infringes upon the cells' ability to perform properly
- Elevated insulin levels
- Heart disease
- High blood sugar, and possibly hyperglycemia or impaired glucose tolerance (IGT)
- Increased cholesterol and triglyceride levels

- Low blood sugar, and possibly hypoglycemia
- Neuropathy (disorders involving nerves)

■ Causes of Chromium Deficiency

- Age
- Antacid use
- Exercise
- High carbohydrate diet
- High intake of refined sugar
- Soil in which food is grown may be low in chromium

■ Factors that Increase Chromium Levels

- Amino acids
- Physical trauma
- Vitamin C

■ Symptoms of Chromium Toxicity

- Lightheadedness
- Rashes

■ Conditions That Can Benefit from Chromium

- High cholesterol levels
- High triglyceride levels
- Hypothyroidism
- Insulin resistance/diabetes
- Osteoporosis
- Sarcopenia (muscle wasting)
- Weight gain
- Yeast overgrowth

■ Recommended Dosage

50 to 200 micrograms daily. Higher dosages may be used to treat a specific disease process, such as those listed above. See your doctor about increasing your chromium intake.

■ Side Effects and Contraindications

If you have compromised kidney function, be sure to speak to your healthcare provider before using a chromium supplement.

■ Food Sources of Chromium

Chromium can be found in the following foods. However, up to 90 percent of the chromium content of food is lost in food processing. If eaten for their chromium content, the following foods should be eaten unprocessed and, most likely, along with chromium supplementation.

This list is reprinted with permission from *Clinical Nutrition: A Functional Approach* by Jeffrey Bland. Foods that contain the most chromium are listed first, followed by foods that contain progressively less chromium. The number to the left of each food describes how many milligrams of chromium are in 100 grams (3.5 ounces) of that food.

112	Brewer's yeast	16	Eggs	8	Navy beans, dry
57	Beef, round	15	Chicken	7	Lettuce
55	Calf's liver	14	Apple	7	Shrimp
42	Whole wheat bread	13	Butter	5	Blueberries
		13	Parsnips	5	Lobster tail
38	Wheat bran	12	Cornmeal	5	Orange
30	Fresh chili	12	Lamb chops	4	Cabbage
30	Rye bread	11	Scallops	4	Green beans
26	Oysters	11	Swiss cheese	4	Mushrooms
24	Potatoes	10	Banana	3	Beer
23	Wheat germ	10	Spinach	3	Strawberries
19	Green pepper	9	Carrots	1	Milk

CYSTEINE

See N-ACETYL CYSTEINE (NAC)

GLUTAMINE

Glutamine is one of the twenty amino acids used to make protein in the body. It is also involved in many metabolic processes. A conditionally essential amino acid, glutamine can be produced by the body but can also become depleted when used in overabundance, such as during intense physical activity or stress.

■ Functions of Glutamine in Your Body

- Balances blood sugar
- Fights cold and flu
- Helps the brain dispose of ammonia
- Improves mental alertness

- Increases energy
- Increases growth hormone
- Is a fueling source for the immune system
- Is a precursor for GABA
- Is an inhibitory neurotransmitter
- Modulates intestinal permeability
- Needed for a healthy gut
- Needed for DHA synthesis
- Needed for the metabolism and maintenance of muscle
- Neutralizes toxins
- Promotes a healthy acid-alkaline balance
- Promotes growth
- Promotes weight loss
- Promotes wound healing and tissue repair
- Protects the body from stress
- Stops food cravings
- Supports glutathione

■ Signs and Symptoms of Glutamine Deficiency

- Anxiety
- Decreased immune system
- Depression
- Insomnia
- Lack of concentration

■ Causes of Glutamine Deficiency

- Intense exercise
- Nutritional deficiencies

■ Conditions That Can Benefit from Glutamine

- Acute pancreatitis/chronic pancreatitis
- ADHD
- After bone marrow transplant to improve recovery
- Alcoholism
- Burn treatment (Used IV or via feeding tube to reduce infections, improve wound healing, and decrease hospitalization time.)
- Crohn's disease
- Cystinuria
- Dysbiosis/leaky gut syndrome
- Enhance energy level in athletes
- HIV to prevent weight loss
- Irritable bowel syndrome (IBS)
- Mucositis secondary to chemotherapy
- Muscle and joint pain caused by the use of Taxol
- Neuropathy
- Prevention of radiation colitis
- Short bowel syndrome
- Sickle cell anemia
- Stomach ulcers

- Stress
- Ulcerative colitis
- Weight gain

▪ Recommended Daily Dosage

500 to 3,000 milligrams daily

▪ Side Effects and Contraindications

If you have a sensitivity to monosodium glutamate (MSG), use glutamine with caution because the body metabolizes glutamine into glutamate. Also use with caution if you take medications for seizures. Use only under a doctor's direction. Until more is known about glutamine supplementation it is recommended that people who have nerve-damaging, chronic neurological diseases, such as ALS and multiple sclerosis, and those who have had recent neurological surgeries limit their intake of supplemental glutamine and/or have glutamine and glutamate levels measured and supplement according to lab levels. Do not use glutamine if you have cirrhosis or hepatic encephalopathy, since it may worsen these conditions. Do not take glutamine if you have manic episodes.

▪ Food Sources

- Asparagus
- Avocados
- Beans
- Broccoli
- Chocolate
- Corn
- Dairy products
- Eggs

- Fish
- Green peas
- Legumes
- Meat
- Nuts
- Oatmeal
- Onion
- Potatoes

- Raisins
- Sesame seeds
- Spinach
- Sunflower seeds
- Swiss chard
- Whey
- Whole grains

MANGANESE

Consuming enough manganese is very important for good health. Most Americans eat enough manganese-containing foods each day and do not need to take supplements. Manganese is a component of some metals and is sometimes inhaled. However, inhaled manganese is not treated by the body the same way ingested manganese is treated. While consumption of manganese has many health benefits, inhaling manganese can cause mental and emotion problems and even brain damage. However, it takes months or years of exposure for this to occur.

Functions of Manganese in Your Body

- Aids in protein digestion and synthesis
- Essential for a healthy nervous system
- Essential for the utilization of vitamins B and C in adrenal health
- Helps with carbohydrate metabolism
- Is a cofactor for enzymes involved in energy production
- Needed for a good immune system
- Needed for brain health
- Needed for the synthesis of cartilage, collagen, and other connective tissue
- Part of the antioxidant defense mechanism
- Required for fatty acid synthesis
- Required for the production of estrogen and progesterone
- Used for bone growth and maintenance
- Used in blood formation

Symptoms of Manganese Deficiency

- Decreased hair and nail growth
- Decreased high-density (good) cholesterol
- Decreased lipid metabolism
- Impaired carbohydrate metabolism
- Impaired growth
- Loss of hair color
- Skeletal problems
- Skin rash

Substances that Lower Your Manganese Levels

- Aluminum
- Phytates in bread and grains (which bind to manganese and prevent it from being bioavailable)

Symptoms of Manganese Toxicity

Like many of the other microminerals, manganese is needed by your body in trace amounts but can be toxic in large quantities. The following list includes the most common symptoms of manganese toxicity.

- Anxiety
- Delusions
- Disorientation
- Emotional liability
- Hallucinations
- Memory loss
- Neurological problems
- Parkinson's disease
- Permanent brain damage

■ Conditions That Can Benefit from Manganese

In addition to the disorders listed below, manganese may be helpful in treating diabetes and epilepsy. However, this has not been proven conclusively.

- Arrhythmias (irregular heart rhythm)
- Arthritic pains
- Back pain
- Premenstrual syndrome (PMS)

■ Recommended Dosage

2.5 to 5 milligrams daily

■ Side Effects and Contraindications

You must be extra cautious consuming manganese if you have gallbladder or liver disease. If you have either of these chronic problems, manganese may be toxic to you. Consult your doctor if you wish to start a manganese regiment but have gallbladder or liver problems.

■ Food Sources of Manganese

The following list is reprinted with permission from Jeffrey Bland's *Clinical Nutrition: A Functional Approach*. Foods that contain the most manganese are listed first, followed by foods that contain progressively less manganese. The number to the left of each food describes how many milligrams of manganese are in 100 grams (3.5 ounces) of that food. Besides the foods listed below, cloves, ginger, thyme, bay leaves, and tea also contain manganese.

3.5	Pecans	1.8	Barley	1.1	Whole wheat
2.8	Brazil nuts	1.3	Buckwheat	0.8	Fresh spinach
2.5	Almonds	1.3	Split peas, dry	0.8	Walnuts

0.7	Peanuts	0.14	Brown rice	0.03	Cantaloupe
0.6	Oats	0.14	Whole wheat bread	0.03	Lamb chops
0.5	Raisins			0.03	Orange
0.5	Rhubarb	0.13	Corn	0.03	Pear
0.5	Turnip greens	0.13	Swiss cheese	0.03	Tomato
0.4	Beet greens	0.11	Cabbage	0.02	Apricot
0.3	Brussels sprouts	0.10	Peach	0.02	Chicken breasts
0.3	Oatmeal	0.09	Butter	0.02	Green beans
0.2	Cornmeal	0.06	Peas	0.02	Whole milk
0.2	Millet	0.06	Tangerine	0.01	Beef liver
0.19	Gorgonzola cheese	0.05	Eggs	0.01	Cucumber
		0.04	Beets	0.01	Halibut
0.16	Carrots	0.04	Coconut	0.01	Scallops
0.15	Broccoli	0.03	Apple		

SELENIUM

Each food's content of selenium, an essential micromineral, depends on the soil in which it is grown. In the United States, the selenium-deficient states are Connecticut, Delaware, Illinois, Indiana, Massachusetts, New York, Ohio, Oregon, Pennsylvania, and Rhode Island. Selenium levels are also low in the District of Columbia. Although selenium supplements have not been proven effective for the prevention of heart disease, a study at The Cleveland Clinic in Ohio suggested that people who lived in states with low selenium content in their soil were three times more likely to die of heart disease than people who lived in states with adequate selenium content in their soil.

■ Functions of Selenium in Your Body

- Helps prevent cancer (due to its role in DNA repair)
- Involved in thyroid function
- May prevent heart disease
- Needed for immune system
- Reduces heavy metal toxicity
- Works with vitamin E as an antioxidant

■ Symptoms of Selenium Deficiency

- Cataracts
- Inflammatory disease
- Loss of pigment in skin and hair
- Low sperm count

- Recurrent infections
- Skeletal muscle problems
- Thyroid enlargement
- Weakness

■ Symptoms of Selenium Toxicity

- Bad breath
- Dry hair
- Fatigue

- Hair loss
- Irritability
- Nervous system problems

■ Causes of Selenium Deficiency

- AIDS
- Autoimmune disease
- Cancer

- Infertility (in males)
- Inflammatory bowel disease
- Thyroid disease

■ Recommended Dosage

200 micrograms once a day

■ Side Effects and Contraindications

Selenium may interfere with the absorption of medications, such as proton-pump inhibitors (PPIs) and histamine blockers.

■ Food Sources of Selenium

The following list is reprinted with permission from Jeffrey Bland's *Clinical Nutrition: A Functional Approach*. Foods that contain the most selenium are listed first, followed by foods that contain progressively less selenium. The number to the left of each food describes how many milligrams of selenium are in 100 grams (3.5 ounces) of that food.

146	Butter	103	Brazil nuts	65	Lobster
141	Smoked herring	77	Scallops	63	Bran
123	Smelt	66	Barley	59	Shrimp
111	Wheat germ	66	Whole wheat bread	57	Red Swiss chard

56	Oats	25	Garlic	4	Radishes
55	Clams	19	Orange juice	4	Grape juice
51	King crab	19	Gelatin	3	Pecans
49	Oysters	19	Beer	2	Hazelnuts
48	Milk	18	Beef liver	2	Almonds
43	Cod	18	Lamb chops	2	Green beans
39	Brown rice	18	Egg yolk	2	Kidney beans
34	Top round steak	12	Mushrooms	2	Onion
		12	Chicken	2	Carrots
30	Lamb	10	Swiss cheese	2	Cabbage
27	Turnips	5	Cottage cheese	1	Orange
26	Molasses	5	Wine		

VITAMIN A

Vitamin A is a fat-soluble vitamin that can be divided into two groups: retinoids (or aldehydes) and carotenoids. Retinoids come from animals and can also be called preformed or active vitamin A because they are already in a form that is usable by the body. Retinal and retinoic acid, which are both found in fish, are included in this grouping. Carotenoids, on the other hand, are found in plants, and are called *provitamins*, which means they are stored in the liver and converted into the usable vitamin as needed. These include beta-carotene, alpha-carotene, and gamma-carotene. Beta-carotene is the most popular and thoroughly studied of the carotenoid varieties. After carotenoids are converted into vitamin A, they react as preformed vitamin A does in the body.

■ Functions of Active Vitamin A in Your Body

- Assists immune function (improves white blood cells, natural killer cells, macrophages, and T and B lymphocytes)
- Needed for the growth and support of the skin
- Needed to detoxify polychlorinated biphenyl (PCB; any of a group of highly toxic compounds often found in industrial waste) and dioxin

- Reduces risk for cancer (esophageal, bladder, stomach, and skin, as well as leukemia and lymphoma)
- Required for vision
- Responsible for healthy mucous membranes
- Strengthens bones during development

Symptoms of Vitamin A Deficiency

- Decreased steroid synthesis
- Dry eyes
- Fatigue
- Hypothyroidism (low thyroid production)
- Increased susceptibility to infections
- Increased susceptibility to vaginal yeast infections
- Night blindness
- Poor tooth and bone function
- Poor wound healing
- Rough, scaly skin

Causes of Vitamin A Deficiency

- Antibiotics
- Cholesterol-lowering medications
- Diabetes
- Decreased intake of vitamin A rich foods
- Laxatives

Substances that Increase Vitamin A Levels

Birth control pills

Symptoms of Vitamin A Toxicity

- Appetite loss
- Bone pain
- Dry skin
- Fatigue
- Hair loss
- Headache
- Irritability
- Joint pain
- Weight loss

Recommended Dosage

5,000 to 10,000 international units daily

■ Side Effects and Contraindications

Excess vitamin A consumption can cause liver damage and even death. If you are taking a high dose, you need to have your doctor measure your calcium and liver enzymes on a regular basis. If you have liver disease, are a smoker, are exposed to asbestos, or are pregnant, you should not consume high doses of vitamin A. Also, a recent study suggested that a daily intake of even 5,000 international units of vitamin A from dietary sources for more than twenty years may increase hip fractures in women.

■ Food Sources of Vitamin A

The following foods are numbered so that the foods that contain the most vitamin A are at the top of the list. As the list proceeds, the foods contain progressively less vitamin A.

1. Liver, lamb	19. Butternut squash	37. Cream, whipped
2. Liver, beef	20. Watercress	38. Peaches
3. Liver, calf	21. Mangos	39. Acorn squash
4. Red chili peppers	22. Sweet red peppers	40. Eggs
5. Dandelion greens	23. Hubbard squash	41. Chicken
6. Liver, chicken	24. Cantaloupe	42. Cherries, sour red
7. Carrots	25. Butter	43. Butterhead lettuce
8. Apricots, dried	26. Endive	44. Asparagus
9. Collard greens	27. Apricots	45. Tomatoes
10. Kale	28. Broccoli spears	46. Green chili peppers
11. Sweet potatoes	29. Whitefish	47. Green peas
12. Parsley	30. Green onions	48. Elderberries
13. Spinach	31. Romaine lettuce	49. Watermelon
14. Turnip greens	32. Papayas	50. Rutabagas
15. Mustard greens	33. Nectarines	51. Brussels sprouts
16. Swiss chard	34. Prunes	52. Okra
17. Beet greens	35. Pumpkin	53. Yellow cornmeal
18. Chives	36. Swordfish	54. Yellow squash

VITAMIN D

The fat-soluble vitamin D is actually not a vitamin (which must be consumed through diet) but a hormone (which is produced in the body). The active form is called 1,25 dihydroxycholecalciferol. Your body produces it after absorbing the sun's rays. I recommend getting sun exposure for ten to fifteen minutes, at least three times a week, if you are depending on the sun for your vitamin D. You can also get vitamin D from food, albeit in smaller doses. Vitamin D-3 comes from red meat and fish; vitamin D-2 comes from plants. In these forms, vitamin D must be metabolized in the body in order to be used by the body, and boron may be needed for the conversion. Vitamin D receptors are located in your bones, pancreas, intestine, kidneys, brain, spinal cord, reproductive organs, thymus, adrenal glands, pituitary gland, and thyroid gland.

▥ Functions of Vitamin D in Your Body

- Aids in the absorption of calcium from the intestinal tract

- Helps the body assimilate phosphorus

- Helps the pancreas release insulin

- Necessary for blood clotting

- Necessary for growth and development of bones and teeth

- Necessary for thyroid function

- Stimulates bone cell mineralization

▥ Symptoms of Vitamin D Deficiency

- Bone disorders (rickets in children or osteomalacia in adults)

- Decreased calcium levels

- Decreased phosphate levels

- Muscle spasms

▥ Causes of Vitamin D Deficiency

- Aging (which causes your body to make less vitamin D from the sun)

- Decreased fat absorption (as a result of short bowel syndrome, sprue, or certain medications)

- Medications (such as phenytoin)

- Prednisone (a steroid that treats cancer and interferes with the conversion of vitamin D to its active form)

- Sunscreen (which prevents vitamin D absorption)

■ Conditions That Can Benefit from Vitamin D

- Autoimmune diseases
- Cancer prevention and treatment
- Cardiovascular disease
- Depression
- Diabetes
- Epilepsy
- Hypertension (high blood pressure)

- Inflammatory conditions
- Migraine headaches
- Multiple sclerosis
- Musculoskeletal pain
- Osteoarthritis
- Polycystic ovary syndrome

■ Recommended Dosage

Consult your medical practitioner, who will conduct lab tests before deciding how much vitamin D you should consume. To get enough vitamin D from the sun's rays, you should expose your face and arms for ten to fifteen minutes, at least three times a week.

■ Side Effects and Contraindications

Vitamin D is stored in the body and can become toxic for some people. At the same time, other people need much higher dosages. Consequently, for dosages above 1,000 international units a day, it is best to consult with your healthcare practitioner. It is necessary to take calcium when taking vitamin D.

■ Food Sources of Vitamin D

The following foods are numbered so that the foods that contain the most vitamin D are at the top of the list. As the list proceeds, the foods contain progressively less vitamin D.

1. Sardines, canned
2. Salmon
3. Tuna
4. Shrimp

5. Butter
6. Sunflower seeds
7. Liver
8. Eggs

9. Milk, fortified
10. Mushrooms
11. Natural cheese

ZINC

Although zinc is a micromineral, and therefore needed by your body only in small quantities, it is very important for your overall physical and mental health. It is used in many enzymatic reactions in your body. Furthermore, there are one hundred enzymes that need zinc as a cofactor. (A cofactor is molecule to which another molecule must bind in order to activate or function.) A recent study revealed that zinc supplementation increases the production of insulin-like growth factor-1 (IGF-1) which is associated with growth and healthier aging. The other functions of zinc are described below.

■ Functions of Zinc in Your Body

- Boosts immune defenses
- Breaks down and metabolizes proteins
- Contributes to a healthy prostate
- Decreases the body's requirement for insulin
- Enhances the biochemical actions of vitamin D
- Essential component of hormones
- Essential for cell division and replication of both DNA and RNA
- Essential for fertility and reproduction
- Has anti-inflammatory effects
- Helps absorption of vitamin A
- Helps assemble proteins inside the cell
- Helps balance blood sugar levels
- Helps stabilize cell membrane and structures within the cell

- Important component of superoxide dismutase, an essential antioxidant
- Improves taste and appetite
- Inhibits the enzyme that reduces levels of the male hormone dihydrotestosterone (DHT)
- Is an antioxidant
- Metabolizes carbohydrates
- Necessary for the proper maintenance of vitamin E
- Needed for the formation of bone and skin
- Promotes thyroid activity
- Related to sexual maturation
- Transports vitamin A to retinas, thereby improving night vision
- Thyroid function (converts certain hormones into their more active forms)

■ Symptoms of Zinc Deficiency

- Acne
- Anemia

- Anorexia
- Behavioral disturbances (such as apathy, confusion, depression, hostility, or irritability)
- Brittle nails
- Craving for sugary foods
- Dandruff
- Decreased ability to taste
- Decreased desire for protein-rich foods
- Decreased sense of smell
- Decreased sexual function
- Delayed sexual maturation
- Diarrhea
- Eczema
- Enlargement of the spleen and liver
- Fatigue
- Frontal headaches
- Growth retardation
- Hair loss
- Immune deficiencies
- Impaired nerve conduction
- Impaired wound healing
- Impotence
- Infertility
- Low sperm count
- Memory impairment
- Negative nitrogen balance
- Nerve damage
- Night blindness
- Poor appetite
- Psoriasis
- Reduced salivation
- Sleep disturbances
- Stretch marks
- White spots on nails

■ Diseases/Disorders that Cause a Predisposition to Zinc Deficiency

- AIDS
- Aging (zinc absorption decreases with age)
- Alcoholism
- Anorexia nervosa
- Celiac disease
- Chronic renal failure
- Cirrhosis
- Cystic fibrosis
- Hemolytic anemia
- Increased calcium ingestion
- Infection
- Inflammatory bowel disease
- Iron supplementation
- Nephrotic syndrome
- Pancreatic insufficiency
- Pancreatitis
- Rheumatoid arthritis

- Short bowel syndrome
- Smoking

- Some diuretics
- Surgery

■ Substances that Decrease Zinc Absorption

- Cortisone
- Coffee and other caffeinated beverages
- Diuretics
- Excess copper

- Foods rich in oxalic acid (such as spinach, sweet potatoes, and rhubarb)
- Foods rich in phytic acid (such as unleavened bread, raw beans, seeds, nuts, and grains)
- Teas containing tannin
- Tetracycline

■ Symptoms of Zinc Toxicity

- Alcohol intolerance
- Anemia
- Decreased immune system
- Dizziness
- Drowsiness

- Hallucinations
- Increased sweating
- Loss of muscular coordination
- Premature heartbeats (heartbeats that occur before the regular heartbeat)

■ Conditions That Can Benefit from Zinc

- Acne
- Anorexia nervosa
- Colds
- Diabetes mellitus
- Eczema
- Enlarged prostate
- Furuncles (bacteria-caused boils)
- Gastric ulcers

- Growth retardation
- Immune function
- Impaired taste sensation
- Infertility
- Macular degeneration (chronic deterioration of retina)
- Rheumatoid arthritis
- Tinnitus

■ Recommended Dosage

25 to 50 milligrams. Try to take zinc at a different time of day from calcium,

copper, iron, and soy, because zinc can interfere with the absorption of these nutrients. When buying zinc supplements, look for zinc picolinate and zinc citrate. These are the two forms of zinc that are best absorbed by your body.

■ Side Effects and Contraindications

Zinc decreases the absorption of fluoroquinolones and tetracyclines, two groups of antibiotics.

■ Food Sources of Zinc

The following list is reprinted with permission from Jeffrey Bland's *Clinical Nutrition: A Functional Approach*. Foods that contain the most zinc are listed first, followed by foods that contain progressively less zinc. The number to the left of each food describes how many milligrams of zinc are in 100 grams (3.5 ounces) of that food. Black pepper, paprika, mustard, chili powder, thyme, and cinnamon are not included on the list but are also high in zinc.

148.7	Fresh oysters	3.0	Walnuts	0.4	Black beans
6.8	Ginger root	2.9	Sardines	0.4	Raw milk
5.6	Ground round steak	2.6	Chicken	0.4	Pork chops
		2.5	Buckwheat	0.4	Corn
5.3	Lamb chops	2.4	Hazel nuts	0.3	Grape juice
4.5	Pecans	1.9	Clams	0.3	Olive oil
4.2	Split peas, dry	1.7	Anchovies	0.3	Cauliflower
4.2	Brazil nuts	1.7	Tuna	0.2	Spinach
3.9	Beef liver	1.7	Haddock	0.2	Cabbage
3.5	Nonfat dry milk	1.6	Green peas	0.2	Lentils
3.5	Egg yolk	1.5	Shrimp	0.2	Butter
3.2	Whole wheat	1.2	Turnips	0.2	Lettuce
3.2	Rye	0.9	Parsley	0.1	Cucumber
3.2	Oats	0.9	Potatoes	0.1	Yams
3.2	Peanuts	0.6	Garlic	0.1	Tangerine
3.1	Lima beans	0.5	Whole wheat bread	0.1	String beans
3.1	Soy lecithin				
3.1	Almonds				

OTHER NUTRIENTS

This section will look at additional nutrients that have not yet been discussed. These nutrients are all important to your nutritional health and overall well-being. Please consult your physician before taking any supplement if you have kidney or liver disease, are pregnant, or are nursing.

BETA GLUCANS

When it comes to *boosting the immune system* by optimizing its response to diseases and infections, beta glucans are very notable to help maintain optimal health. They are found in baker's yeast (Saccharomyces cerevisiae), shiitake mushrooms, and cereal grains such as barley, oats, rye, and wheat.

Functions of Beta Glucans in Your Body

- Anti-cancer properties
- Is an immune-stimulating agent, acts through the activation of macrophages and NK cell cytotoxicity
- May inhibit tumor growth in the promotion stage
- Anti-angiogenesis (may prevent tumor metastasis)
- Acts as an adjuvant to cancer chemotherapy and radiotherapy by restoring hematopoiesis following bone marrow injury
- Antigenotoxic activity (chemical agents that damage the genetic information within a cell causing mutations)
- Antimutagenic activity (reduces rate of mutations)
- Anti-inflammatory
- Antioxidant
- Blood sugar regulation
- Builds the immune system by activating the anti-microbial immune response
- Stimulates the activity of macrophages which increases phagocytosis, selective cytokine release, and oxidative degranulation
- Activates T cell medicated immunity

- Stimulates lymphocytes that bind to tumors or viruses and release chemicals to destroy it

- Acts on several immune receptors including Dectin-1, complement receptor (CR3) and TLR-2/6

- Triggers a group of immune cells including macrophages, neutrophils, monocytes, natural killer cells, and dendritic cells.

- Decreases the risk of infection

- Enhances antibiotic efficacy in animals infected with antibiotic-resistant bacteria

- Enhances tumor necrosis factor alpha (TNF-alpha)

- Has positive effects on the skin: anti-wrinkle activity, anti-ultraviolet light activity, wound healing, and moisturizing effects as well as providing structure and elasticity to the skin.

- Lowers cholesterol

- Prophylactic administration of beta-glucan was found to positively affect levels of the antioxidant enzymes catalase and superoxide dismutase, moderate tissue-damaging cytokines, and assist in ameliorating microbial imbalance.

■ Recommended Daily Dosage

Saccharomyces cerevisiae—250 mg to 500 mg once a day NOT with a meal. Usually, it is suggested to take first thing in the morning or last thing at night with 8 ounces of water. You can take up to two capsules a day.

■ Conditions That Can Benefit from Beta Glucans

- Aids in treatment of antibiotic-resistant infections

- Allergies

- Anti-aging skin care

- Builds the immune system

- Fights against cancer (antioxidant, antimutagenic, antigenotoxic)

- Hematopoiesis (process of creating new blood cells from stem cells) following radiation or other bone marrow insults

- Hypercholesterolemia (high cholesterol)

- Inflammatory diseases

- Insulin resistance/diabetes

- Traveler's diarrhea

■ Side Effects and Contraindications

Do not use if you have an allergy to mushrooms, wheat, rye, oats, barley, or other cereal grains.

CARNOSINE

Carnosine is an amino acid that is formed when a beta-alanine molecule and a histidine molecule join together. Stored in the brain, heart, and muscles, it protects the body from glycation. Studies have shown that carnosine is effective against cross-linking and the formation of advanced glycation end products (AGE) and it also decreases free radical production. In fact, one study showed carnosine was the only antioxidant to significantly protect cellular chromosomes from oxidative damage. Carnosine has been shown to inhibit glycation in eye lens protein and furthermore, carnosine is a potent copper-zinc chelating agent that can inhibit the cross-linking of beta-amyloid that leads to brain cell plaque formation. Do not confuse this nutrient with the similar-sounding amino acid carnitine. Carnosine has likewise been shown to protect against influenza much like chicken soup and chicken breast extracts that are rich in carnosine and its derivative anserine.

■ Functions of Carnosine in Your Body

- Acts as an antioxidant
- Attenuation of the effects of cytokines and chemokines
- Binds metal ions that cause tissue damage
- Blocks the aging effects of glycation
- Has anti-inflammatory action
- Has direct interaction with nitric oxide
- Helps maintain memory
- Inhibits cytotoxic nitric oxide-induced proinflammatory conditions
- Protects against peroxynitrate damage
- Protects muscle tissue from lactic acid
- Provides a barrier against influenza viral infection
- Regulates levels of copper and zinc

■ Signs and Symptoms of Carnosine Deficiency

- Cataract formation
- Cognitive decline

- Dry eyes

- Hypertension (high blood pressure)

Causes of Carnosine Deficiency

- Dietary deficiencies in nutrients that make beta-alanine and histidine

- Decreased intake in foods that make carnosine

Conditions That Can Benefit from Carnosine

- Aging

- Alzheimer's disease

- Atherosclerosis

- Autism

- Brain injury

- Cataracts

- Diabetes mellitus

- Dry eyes

- Hypertension

- Skin aging

- Stroke

- Wound healing

Recommended Daily Dosage

1,000 to 2,000 milligrams daily in people with normal renal function. Carnosine can also be used as eye drops for dry eyes.

Side Effects and Contraindications

Do not supplement if you have kidney or liver disease without consulting your healthcare provider. Also, be aware that if you take too much carnosine it can result in hyperactivity.

Food Sources

- Beef

- Chicken

- Pork

COLOSTRUM

Colostrum, a nutrient with immune-enhancing benefits, is secreted by humans and animals in breast milk. It can also be taken as a supplement. Furthermore, colostrum contains protein and carbohydrate, vitamins and minerals, along with cytokines, which include IL-1-beta, IL-6, trypsin inhibitors, protease inhibitors and oligosaccharides. In addition, colostrum contains several types of growth factors.

Functions of Colostrum in Your Body

- Antibacterial and antiviral effects
  - Clostridium difficile
  - Cryptosporidium parvum
  - E. Coli
  - H. Pylori
  - Rotavirus
  - Shigella flexneuri
  - Streptococcus mutans
- Anti-inflammatory
- Antioxidant
- Immunomodulatory
- Immune builder
- Improves gut permeability
- Reduces nonsteroidal anti-inflammatory drug (NSAID)-induced intestinal damage

Conditions That Can Benefit from Colostrum

- Chemotherapy-induced mouth ulcers
- Food allergies
- Improves physical performance and preservation of muscle mass
- Infection prevention
  - Decreases incidence of upper respiratory tract infections
  - Influenza
  - Rotavirus
  - Shigella infection
- Infection treatment
  - HIV infection
  - Rotavirus
- Inflammatory bowel disease
- May improve blood sugar
- May also protect the stomach and bowel from damage caused by anti-inflammatory medications
- Short bowel syndrome
- Systemic inflammatory response syndrome (SIRS)
- Wound healing

Recommended Daily Dosage

The following are recommended daily dosages per clinical condition.

- Diarrhea caused by HIV: 10 grams daily
- Diarrhea due to rotavirus: 100 mL three times a day for three days. Colostrum must be from cows immunized with the four serotypes of human rotavirus to be effective
- Improving athletic performance: 10 grams daily

- Increasing growth factors: 20 grams daily

- Prevention of NSAID-induced GI damage: 125 mL three times a day

- Prevention of URI: 60 grams daily

Side Effects and Contraindications

None known

GLUTATHIONE

Glutathione is a *tripeptide*—a compound composed of three amino acids—that is made of cysteine, glutamic acid, and glycine. It is responsible for the health of most of the cells in your body. Around the age of forty, your glutathione levels begin to diminish, and you may need to begin taking it as a supplement.

Functions of Glutathione in Your Body

- Decreases sugar cravings

- Displaces glutamate from its binding site

- Enhances liver and brain detoxification of toxic chemicals and heavy metals

- Helps to recycle other antioxidants, such as vitamins C and E

- Involved in protein and prostaglandin (fatty acid compounds) synthesis

- Is a neuromodulator (transmits information between neurons)

- Is a neurotransmitter

- Is a powerful antioxidant

- Part of amino acid transport

- Stimulates production of interleukin 1 and 2, which help regulate your immune system

- Used in DNA synthesis and repair

Symptoms of Glutathione Deficiency

- Faster progression of human immunodeficiency virus (HIV)

- Hemolytic anemia (destruction of red blood cells)

- Immune disorders

Causes of Glutathione Deficiency

- Acetaminophen

- Cigarette smoking

- Excessive intake of alcohol
- Overly processed chemical-laden foods (such as luncheon meats that contain nitrites or nitrates)

Nutrients that Increase Glutathione Levels

- Alpha-lipoic acid
- Glutamine
- Methionine
- Milk thistle
- S-adenosyl methionine (SAMe)
- Vitamin C
- Vitamin E
- Whey protein

Recommended Dosage

Taking 500 to 3,000 milligrams of n-acetyl cysteine (NAC) daily will increase your glutathione levels.

Most forms of glutathione are not effective if taken by mouth because they are broken down by digestive enzymes. Instead, they can be given to you by your physician intravenously. Glutathione can be taken orally, however, if in a specific form called liposomal glutathione. This amino acid linkage is not broken down by digestive enzymes.

Side Effects and Contraindications

The cysteine in NAC can precipitate and cause kidney stones to form. Take extra vitamin C with NAC to avoid this. Also, if you are taking NAC for prolonged periods of time, you may need to take extra copper and zinc. NAC can bind these minerals and make them unavailable for usage in your body.

Food Sources of Glutathione

- Asparagus
- Avocado
- Fish
- Meat
- Walnuts

SULFORAPHANE

Sulforaphane is an isothiocyanate occurring in a stored form as glucoraphanin in cruciferous vegetables, such as cabbage, cauliflower, kale, broccoli, and especially in broccoli sprouts. It is generated by damage to the plant and is involved in protecting the plant from insect predators.

Glucoraphanin requires the plant enzyme myrosinase for converting it into sulforaphane. Sulforaphane is metabolized through the mercapturic acid pathway, being conjugated with glutathione and it undergoes further biotransformation, yielding metabolites. It also produces heat shock proteins.

▣ Functions of Sulforaphane in Your Body

- Active against H. pylori (a bacteria that can attack the lining of the stomach)

- Ameliorates bronchoconstrictor effects (narrowing of the airways in the lungs)

- Anti-inflammatory

- Antineoplastic (anti-cancer) and chemo-preventive by regulating the expression of more than 200 cytoprotective genes

- Antioxidant

- Antiviral

- Decreases expression of cyclin D2, surviving, and DNA synthesis

- Decreases transcription of nuclear factor kB and antiapoptotic proteins

- Increases natural killer cell (NK) cell production

- Increases Nrf2 gene activity which coordinates activity of detoxifying genes

- Interferes with genome compacting (by inhibition of histone deacetylases and disrupts Hsp90 complexes, which cause cell cycle arrest, mitosis interruption, activation of caspases, and mitochondria depolarization)

- Potent inducer of phase II enzymes in the liver

▣ Conditions That Can Benefit from Sulforaphane

- ARDS (may have prophylactic and curative effect)

- Asthma

- Autism

- Cancer prevention and therapy

- Cardiovascular disease prevention

- Hepatitis C

- HIV (Inhibits HIV infection of macrophages through Nrf2)

- Influenza

- Insulin resistance/diabetes

- Osteoporosis

- SARS-CoV-2 (may have prophylactic and therapeutic effect)

■ Recommended Daily Dosage

Dosing will depend on the active component contained in the supplement. Most common dose is 10 to 30 mg twice a day.

■ Side Effects and Contraindications

- No side effects have been reported

- Sulforaphane may interact with medications changed by the liver (cyto-chrome P450 1A2 (CYP1A2) substrates. Therefore, use with caution in patients taking medications that clear through the liver.

THERAPIES THAT DECREASE INFLAMMATION

This section covers natural ways to lower inflammation in your body and to protect yourself from disease. Without the possible side effects that exist with anti-inflammatory drugs, these therapies have the potential to be effective in treating or protecting against inflammation.

ALOE VERA

Aloe vera (*Aloe barbadensis*) is usually utilized for skin burns, infections, and wounds and applied as a topical ointment, gel, or spray. The gel-like center of the plant's leaves is extracted and used for this purpose. It can also be taken orally, although this has been studied less than its topical treatment. The liquid found in between the gel and outer leaf can be dried and ingested.

■ Functions of Aloe Vera in Your Body

- Antibiotic and antiseptic properties (kills germs and bacteria)
- Encourages healing
- Improves ability to heal from wounds
- Reduces inflammation
- Relieves pain from certain skin conditions
- Strengthens immune system
- Works as a laxative

■ Conditions That Topical Aloe Vera Can Treat or Protect Against

- Aphthous stomatitis
- Burns
- Dandruff
- Eczema
- Genital herpes
- Herpes simplex
- Psoriasis
- Skin infections
- Various wounds

■ Conditions That Oral Aloe Vera Can Treat or Protect Against

- AIDS
- Asthma
- Constipation
- Diabetes
- Inflammation
- Inflammatory bowel disease

- Peptic ulcer disease

■ Recommended Dosage

- As a topical cream, Aloe vera can be applied liberally with no side effects.

- When taken orally, up to 150 milligrams of Aloe vera can usually be taken without causing any discomfort.

■ Side Effects and Contraindications

There are no noted side effects when using Aloe vera as a topical cream, but it should not be used on deep surgical wounds. When taken orally, Aloe vera can cause diarrhea and nausea. In addition, abusing Aloe vera (orally) can result in dangerous electrolyte imbalances such as low potassium levels.

AMERICAN SKULLCAP

Skullcap may sound like the hat but it's actually a medicinal plant that's long been used for healing purposes. This medicinal plant references two herbs: American skullcap (*Scutellaria lateriflora*) and Chinese skullcap (*Scutellaria baicalensis*). Each are therapies for different medical conditions. This section refers to American Skullcap (Scuttelaria lateriflora). It is a member of the mint family.

■ Functions of American Skullcap in Your Body

- Anxiolytic (anti-anxiety)
- Decreases inflammation
- Immune modulation
- Lowers blood sugar
- Lowers cholesterol

■ Recommended Daily Dosage

Dose depends on your age, kidney function, and weight.

■ Side Effects and Contraindications

Make sure you purchase pharmaceutical grade American skullcap since in the past it has been contaminated with germander (Teucrium) which is part of a group of plants that can cause liver dysfunction. Do not use with herbs that have a sedating effect: valerian, catnip, and kava. Use with caution if you are diabetic since it lowers blood sugar. You may need less medication or other therapies for your blood sugar when taking American skullcap. This herb should not be used during pregnancy or if you are breast breastfeeding. American skullcap can increase the effect of medications that have a sedating effect, such as barbiturates, benzodiazepine, medications for insomnia, tricyclic antidepressants, and alcohol.

High doses of American skullcap can cause any of the following symptoms:

- Giddiness
- Seizures
- Irregular heartbeat
- Stupor
- Mental confusion
- Twitching

■ Conditions That Can Benefit from American Skullcap

- Allergies
- Insomnia
- Anxiety
- Insulin resistance
- Depression
- Nervous tension
- Epilepsy
- Parkinson's disease
- Heart disease
- Skin infections
- Hypercholesterolemia (high cholesterol)
- Spasms
- Stroke
- Inflammation

BOSWELLIA

Boswellia (*Boswellia serrata*) has been used to treat inflammatory conditions for many centuries. *Boswellia serrata* possesses monoterpenes, diterpenes, triterpenes, tetracyclic triterpenic acids and four major pentacyclic triterpenic acids which are responsible for inhibition of pro-inflammatory enzymes. It inactivates NFkappaB (a protein complex that controls transcription of DNA, cytokine production and cell survival) and down regulates TNF-alpha (a protein manufactured by white blood cells that when overproduced can lead to disease where the immune system acts against healthy tissues) and decreases proinflammatory cytokines. In addition, Boswellia decreases the activity of human leukocyte elastase (HLE), an inflammatory enzyme associated with rheumatoid arthritis, pulmonary emphysema, cystic fibrosis, chronic bronchitis, and acute respiratory distress syndrome.

■ Functions of Boswellia in Your Body

- Cytotoxic and antitumor properties
- Lowers blood sugar
- Lowers cholesterol
- Modules immune system
- Raises HDL (good cholesterol)
- Strong anti-inflammatory agent

■ Conditions That Can Benefit from Boswellia

- Acute respiratory distress syndrome (ARDS)
- Asthma
- Cancer
- Chronic bronchitis
- Cystic fibrosis
- Hypercholesterolemia (elevated cholesterol)
- Insulin resistance/diabetes
- Irritable bowel disease
- Osteoarthritis
- Peptic ulcer disease
- Psoriasis
- Rheumatoid arthritis

■ Recommended Daily Dosage

The most common choice is to take Boswellia 300 to 500 mg BID to TID of an extract standardized to contain 30 to 40 percent Boswellic acids. The complete effect may take several weeks.

■ Side Effects and Contraindications

Do not us Boswellia if you are pregnant. It may stimulate blood flow in the uterus and pelvis and therefore may increase menstrual flow and may induce miscarriage. Boswellia may also interact with NSAIDs including aspirin. Possible side effects include: nausea, acid reflux, diarrhea, and skin rashes.

CAYENNE PEPPER

Cayenne (*Capsicum annuum* or red pepper) is popular as both a whole pepper and as a hot cooking spice. However, cayenne also has a number of healing abilities, including the potential to improve the entire circulatory and digestive systems. Capsicum also contains vitamins A and C, flavonoids, and carotenoids. Furthermore, capsaicin stimulates nerve endings, so they release substance P which transmits pain signals to the brain. When a nerve ending has released all of its substance P reserves, pain signals are no longer sent to the brain until substance P has been replenished. Pain then decreases or resolves. Cayenne is very potent and, consequently, it is very important to wash your hands after using it, as well as to avoid contact between it and eyes, open wounds, or mucous membranes. If you hard time getting cayenne off of the skin, apply vinegar to the skin.

■ Functions of Cayenne in Your Body

- Anti-inflammatory actions
- Diminishes awareness of pain
- Helps the body digest
- Improves blood flow and circulation
- Is an antioxidant
- Lowers blood sugar
- Lowers LDL (bad) cholesterol

■ Symptoms of Cayenne Toxicity

- Gastroenteritis
- Kidney damage
- Liver damage

■ Conditions That Can Benefit from Cayenne Pepper

- Cluster headaches
- Cramps
- Heart disease
- Indigestion
- Inflammation
- Insulin resistance/diabetes
- Irregular heart rhythm (has antiarrhythmic properties)
- Nerve pain
- Obesity
- Osteoarthritis
- Peripheral neuropathy (numbness and tingling of the extremities) due to diabetes
- Poor appetite
- Psoriasis
- Rheumatoid arthritis
- Shingles
- Sore throat

■ Recommended Daily Dosage

- As a capsule: 20 to 100 milligrams, three times a day.

- As a topical cream: Apply a thin
coat three or four times a day
for three weeks. Do not apply to
broken skin.

■ Side Effects and Contraindications

Oral Cayenne

- As a capsule: may cause nausea or vomiting if taken in too high a dose.

- Capsaicin capsules may cause stomach irritation. Use with caution if you have heartburn or ulcers.

- Individuals who are allergic to latex, bananas, kiwi, chestnuts, and avocado may also be allergic to cayenne.

- Pregnant women should not take cayenne as a supplement.

- Cayenne does pass into breast milk, so nursing mothers should avoid cayenne as a supplement.

- Cayenne may increase the risk of developing a cough if you are on an ace inhibitor. Listed are some of the ace inhibitors that are prescribed worldwide. If you do not know if you are on an ace inhibitor, then speak to your healthcare provider.
  - Captopril
  - Elaropril
  - Fosinopril
  - Lisinopril

- Capsaicin may make aspirin less effective as a pain reliever. It may also increase the risk of bleeding associated with aspirin.

- It increases stomach acid so cayenne may make antacids and PPI's less effective medications or over-the-counter products.

- Capsaicin may increase the risk of bleeding associated with blood-thinning medications and herbs such as ginkgo, ginseng, ginger, and garlic.

- Capsaicin lowers blood sugar levels and may increase the risk of hypoglycemia (low blood sugar) in people taking blood sugar lowering medications.

- Use cayenne with caution in patients on theophylline since regular use of red pepper may increase absorption of this medication.

Topical Cayenne

- As a topical cream it may cause burning or itching in some individuals. This usually subsides after several uses. If it does not, then discontinue use. Test the capsaicin cream on a small area of your skin first before applying it to large areas.

- Do not use capsaicin with a heating pad, and do not apply capsaicin cream immediately before or after a hot shower.

CHINESE SKULLCAP

There are two forms of skullcap. This section refers to Chinese skullcap which is also known as Baikal skullcap (*Scutellaria baicalensis*). It is a member of the mint family. This herb has been used in China for many years to treat a number of health problems, including high blood pressure, hepatitis, constipation, and various viruses. Chinese skullcap is, however, particularly well known for treating conditions associated with inflammation. Its anti-inflammatory qualities are from the isoflavones it contains—baicalein, baicalin, and wogonin.

■ Functions of Chinese Skullcap in Your Body

- Antifibrotic (inhibits fibrosis and lipid peroxidation caused by bile duct ligation or carbon tetrachloride)
- Anxiolytic (antianxiety)
- Decreases inflammation since it inhibits COX-2
- Immune modulation
- Inhibits histamine response
- Liver protective
- Lowers blood pressure
- Lowers blood sugar
- Lowers cholesterol
- Lowers triglycerides

■ Conditions That Can Benefit from Chinese Skullcap

- Allergies
- Antibacterial agent
- Antiemetic
- Antiviral agent (hepatitis C)
- Anxiety
- Cancer (adjunct to chemotherapy)
- Chronic active hepatitis (combined with other herbal therapies)
- Epilepsy (combined with other herbal therapies)

- Fungus
- Gingivitis
- Headaches
- Hypercholesterolemia (high cholesterol)
- Hypertension (high blood pressure)
- Hypertriglyceridemia (high triglycerides)
- Infections (antifungal and antiviral)
- Inflammation
- Insulin resistance
- Liver fibrosis (combined with other herbal therapies)
- Neuroprotective
- Noise induced hearing loss (mouse model)
- Ulcers

■ Recommended Daily Dosage

Dose depends on your age, kidney function, and weight.

■ Side Effects and Contraindications

Do not use with herbs that have a sedating effect: valerian, catnip, and kava. Use with caution if you are diabetic since it lowers blood sugar. You may need less medication or other therapies for your blood sugar when taking American skullcap.

This herb should not be used during pregnancy or if you are breast breast-feeding. Also, do not use Chinese skullcap if you have stomach problems or dysfunction of your spleen.

Chinese skullcap can interfere with the following medications: cyclosporine, ciprofloxacin, doxorubicin, and it may increase the risk of bleeding if you are taking warfarin. In addition, there have been reported cases of interstitial pneumonia and acute respiratory failure. This risk is increased in the elderly, with duration of usage, and if you are taking the drug interferon.

CURCUMIN

Curcumin is a phytonutrient derived from the spice turmeric (*Curcuma longa*) that has been used for over 4,000 years. Turmeric, the main element of curry, is a member of the ginger family. Curcumin has many medicinal benefits. It has a long history of relieving inflammation by inhibiting certain enzymes and other substances within the inflammatory pathway. It can lower LDL (bad) cholesterol and total cholesterol. Curcumin may also prove to have an anti-cancer effect. Furthermore, clinical trials have shown that curcumin may help maintain cognition and treat inflammatory bowel diseases. It has also been shown to reduce both duodenal and gastric ulcers. Curcumin is also used in cosmetics, as a flavoring agent for food, and for food coloring giving it a nice yellow color.

■ Functions of Curcumin in Your Body

- Anti-inflammatory
- Antioxidant

- Improves digestion
- Lowers blood sugar

■ Conditions That Can Benefit from Curcumin

- Cancer
- Cognition decline/Alzheimer's disease
- Dyspepsia (indigestion)
- Indigestion (relieves gas and bloating)
- Insulin resistance/diabetes
- Irritable bowel syndrome

- Lowers c-reactive protein
- Multiple sclerosis
- Osteoarthritis
- Parkinson's disease
- Tropical pancreatitis
- Ulcerative colitis
- Uveitis

■ Recommended Daily Dosage

400 to 600 mg three times a day.

■ Side Effects and Contraindications

If you are pregnant or breast feeding, do not take turmeric supplements. Because curcumin may act like a blood thinner, discontinue its use two weeks before surgery. Also consult your healthcare provider before taking if you are on a drug that is a blood thinner. Do not use if you have gallstones since it stimulates the gallbladder to produce bile. Curcumin lowers blood sugar, if you are taking nutrients or medications for insulin resistance or diabetes, check your blood sugar on a regular basis especially if you are using this herb. Curcumin can interfere with drugs that decrease stomach acid since this herb can increase the production of stomach acid. Therefore, do not use if you have peptic ulcers.

FEVERFEW

Feverfew (*Tanacetum parthenium*) is an herb used to treat migraine headaches. This herb needs to be taken for at least a month to effectively prevent migraine headaches. Feverfew, furthermore, reduces inflammation, decreases histamine release, and reduces fever. The name comes from the Latin word *febrifugia*, "fever reducer." The plant contains several products, but the active components probably include one or more of the sesquiterpene lactones. Other active constituents include flavonoid glycosides and pinenes.

■ Functions of Feverfew in Your Body

- Anti-cancer
- Anti-inflammatory
- Anti-spasmodic
- Bone regulation
- Emmenagogue (stimulates menstrual flow)
- Heart protective
- Immunomodulatory (anti-bacterial, anti-fungal, anti-TB)
- Inhibits histamine release
- Inhibits muscle spasm
- Inhibits serotonin release and binding
- Sedative
- Tranquilizing

■ Conditions That Can Benefit from Feverfew

- Allergies
- Anemia
- Arthritis
- Asthma
- Cancer
- Common cold
- Decreases vascular smooth muscles
- Diarrhea
- Dizziness
- Earache
- Fever reduction
- Infertility
- Insect bites
- Irregular menstrual cycles
- Migraine headaches
- Muscle tension
- Nausea and vomiting
- Osteoporosis
- Prevention of miscarriage
- Psoriasis
- Rheumatoid arthritis

- Stomachache
- Tinnitus (ringing in the ears)
- Toothache
- Upset stomach

■ Recommended Daily Dosage

For migraine headaches: 100 to 300 mg, up to 4 times daily, standardized to contain 0.2 to 0.4% parthenolides.

■ Side Effects and Contraindications

If you are allergic to plants in the daisy family, such as chamomile, yarrow, or ragweed, you should not take Feverfew. This herb also has the potential to interact with anticoagulant drugs such as Coumadin and similar medications. Therefore, use only under a healthcare provider's direction if you are taking a blood thinner. One study showed that patients that switched to placebo after taking feverfew for several years experienced the following symptoms: headaches, insomnia, joint pain, nervousness, poor sleep patterns, stiffness, tension, tiredness, along with muscle and joint stiffness. This phenomenon is called "post-feverfew" syndrome. Therefore, do not abruptly stop taking feverfew if you have used it for more than one week. Possible side effects of feverfew include:

- Abdominal pain
- Diarrhea
- Gas
- Indigestion
- Mouth ulcers
- Nausea
- Nervousness
- Vomiting

In addition, feverfew can cause inflammation of the oral mucosa and tongue, with lip swelling, and loss of taste particularly if the leaves are chewed. Contact dermatitis (rash) has been seen with this plant. The use of feverfew is contraindicated in pregnancy. It is also not recommended for breastfeeding women or for use in children.

FISH OIL

See Omega-3-Fatty Acid in Part 2, page 000.

GINGER

Ginger (*Zingiber officinale*) has been used for culinary and medicinal purposes for thousands of years. The root (or rhizomes) of the ginger plant can be consumed fresh or cooked; powdered and used as a flavoring or to make tea; infused into an oil; or juiced. Medicinal forms of ginger include teas, tinctures, capsules, and lozenges.

Ginger has been extensively studied and found to contain many beneficial substances. Of these, the best known are gingerols and shogaols, both of which exhibit a host of biological activities.

Functions of Ginger in Your Body

- Accelerates gastric emptying and stimulates stomach contractions
- Balances the immune system
- Decreases dizziness
- Decreases nausea and vomiting
- Enhances wound healing
- Has anti-ulcer activity
- Improves heart function
- Improves insulin sensitivity (blood sugar)
- Is an antihistamine
- Is an antioxidant
- Is antifungal
- Is anti-inflammatory
- Is antimicrobial
- Is antiviral
- Lowers blood pressure
- Prevents platelets from sticking together and forming blood clots
- Protects healthy tissues from anti-cancer drugs
- Protects the kidneys
- Protects the liver
- Reduces anxiety
- Relaxes smooth muscle cells
- Stimulates the flow of saliva, bile, and gastric secretions

Conditions That Can Benefit from Ginger

- Allergies
- Asthma
- Indigestion
- Insulin resistance/diabetes
- Mastitis (inflammation of breast tissue)
- Menstrual cramps
- Migraine headache (prevention and treatment)
- Motion sickness
- Nausea
- Osteoarthritis

- Post-exercise induced muscle pain
- Rheumatoid arthritis
- Stomach cramps

- Ulcerative colitis
- Weight gain
- Wounds

■ Recommended Dosage

500 milligrams twice a day. Do not take more than 4 grams of ginger a day, including food sources.

■ Side Effects and Contraindications

Ginger can act as a blood thinner. If you have a bleeding disorder or are taking a medication or supplement that may thin your blood, do not take this supplement. If you are planning to have surgery, discontinue this herbal therapy two weeks before the procedure. Speak to your healthcare provider or pharmacist to learn if any drugs you're taking might make it unwise to take ginger supplements.

It is rare to have side effects from ginger, but some may occur. Taking ginger in capsule form or with meals may help you avoid the following side effects:

- Diarrhea
- Heartburn
- Stomach upset

Used topically, ginger may cause contact dermatitis. If this occurs, discontinue use.

GREEN TEA

Although green tea has been popular in Eastern countries, such as China, India, and Japan, for much of recorded history, it has also become increasingly popular in the Western world. Recognized for its varied medicinal benefits, green tea is particularly praised for its high content of antioxidants. It is from the Camellia sinensis plant, as are black tea and oolong tea, but is steamed rather than fermented. This allows it to retain its healthful qualities, unlike the other two teas. Green tea can be taken as a capsule or drank as a tea.

■ Functions of Green Tea in Your Body

- Antibacterial effect
- Antiviral effect

- Chelates iron, zinc, and copper
- Decreases leptin levels

- Improves alertness
- Improves heart health
- Inhibits growth of cancerous cells
- Inhibits platelet aggregation (clumping of platelets which increases your risk of heart disease)
- Is an antioxidant
- Kills unhealthy bacteria in both body and mouth

- Lowers blood pressure
- Lowers LDL cholesterol (bad cholesterol)
- Lowers triglyceride levels
- May encourage weight loss
- Regulates blood sugar level
- Restricts growth of unhealthy blood clots

■ Conditions That Can Benefit from Green Tea

- Allergies
- Amyloidosis (when heart involvement is present)
- Arthritis
- Asthma
- Beta-thalassemia (due to iron chelating effect)
- Cancer (prevention and treatment of cancers including bladder, breast, colon, liver, lung, pancreas, prostate, skin, small intestine, and stomach)
- Cardiovascular disease
- Dental caries and gingivitis
- Depression

- Diabetes
- Diarrhea
- Genital warts
- Hypercholesterolemia (high cholesterol)
- Hypertriglyceridemia (high triglycerides)
- Infection
- Irritable bowel syndrome (IBS)
- May inhibit kidney stone formation
- Obesity
- Ulcerative colitis
- Weight loss (studies are mixed on efficacy)

■ Recommended Daily Dosage

Studies were done on 3 to 10 cups of green tea a day. Do not take directly with iron supplements since the tannins in green tea may bind to iron and decrease its absorption.

■ Side Effects and Contraindications

• Green tea contains caffeine, therefore some drinkers experience insomnia or restlessness. However, the amount of caffeine contained in a glass of tea is minimal compared to that in coffee or soda.

• Some drinkers of green tea have had allergic reactions. The most common effects experienced were anxiety; constipation or diarrhea; headache; loss of appetite; and nausea.

• Due to its caffeine content, use with caution if you have high blood pressure, cardiac arrhythmias (irregular heart rhythm), anxiety, psychiatric disorders, insomnia, or severe liver disease.

• Green tea has been shown to reduce blood levels of lithium making lithium less effective. Consult your healthcare provider if you are on lithium before intaking more than one cup of green tea a day.

• Do not use green tea if you are taking a MAO inhibitor.

• Caffeine from green tea, and phenylpropanolamine, used in many over-the-counter and prescription cough and cold medications and weight loss products, may cause mania and high blood pressure.

• Caffeinated green tea may interact with a number of medications:

• Acetaminophen	• Fluvoxamine
• Adenosine	• Methotrexate
• Beta-lactam antibiotics	• Mexiletine
• Carbamazepine	• Phenobarbital
• Clozapine	• Quinolone antibiotics
• Dipyridamole	• Theophylline
• Estrogen	• Verapamil

N-ACETYL CYSTEINE

N-acetyl cysteine (NAC) is derived from the sulfur containing amino acid cysteine. Amino acids are building blocks of proteins. Furthermore, NAC is a glutathione precursor and has been used in therapeutic practices for decades, as a mucolytic agent and for the treatment of numerous disorders including acetaminophen overdose. N-acetyl cysteine also has antiviral effects.

■ Functions of N-Acetyl Cysteine in Your Body

- Alters the microvascular tone to increase the blood flow and oxygen delivery to the liver and other vital organs
- Antioxidant
- Anti-inflammatory
  - Affects release of IL-1B, IL-8, and TNF-alpha, IL-6
  - Decreases production of pro-inflammatory cytokines
  - Inhibits activation of oxidant sensitive pathways including transcription factor NF-kappaB
  - Inhibits mitogen activated protein kinase p38
- Anti-viral effects
  - Inhibits replication of season influenza
  - Reduces the production of pro-inflammatory molecules (CXCL8, CXCL10, CCL5 and interleukin-6 (IL-6))
- Reduces monocyte migration
- Binds to toxic metabolites
- Direct reactive oxygen species (ROS) scavenger regulating the redox status in the cells
- Improves brain functional connectivity
- Increases mitochondrial ATP production (energy production)
- Increases oxygen delivery to tissues
- Inhibits oxidative stress
- Lowers lipoprotein a (risk factor for heart disease)
- Mucolytic agent
- Replenishes glutathione reserves by providing cysteine which is needed for glutathione production

■ Recommended Daily Dosage

- The dosage of NAC varies according to route of administration and clinical usage.
  - Bronchitis: 200 mg twice a day to 200 mg three times a day
  - Influenza: 600 mg twice a day for up to 3 months
  - IV: see healthcare provider
  - Inhaled: see healthcare provider

■ Side Effects and Contraindications

- NAC can cause a false positive result for urine ketones.

- Oral NAC can cause any or all of the following symptoms:
  - Nausea and vomiting. Use with caution if you GI ulcers or varices.
  - NAC can cause constipation, diarrhea, flatus, and gastroesophageal reflux.
  - NAC may rarely cause headaches, fever, rashes, drowsiness, low blood pressure, and hepatic issues.
- NAC has an unpleasant odor that some people may find offensive.
- IV NAC may cause the following symptoms:
  - It can cause rate related anaphylactoid reactions in up to 18 percent of individuals that is not seen with oral administration.
  - NAC used IV can cause a spurious increase in INR (blood clotting study) which normalizes when it is discontinued.
  - Nausea, vomiting, diarrhea, or constipation
  - Rarely it may cause headache fever, rash, drowsiness, low blood pressure, and liver issues.
- Inhaled NAC may cause the following symptoms:
  - Chest tightness
  - Clamminess
  - Drowsiness
  - Runny nose
  - Swelling in the mouth
- NAC has not been adequately studied in women that are pregnant or breastfeeding. Therefore, do not use in these conditions.
- Do not use if you are allergic to cysteine.
- Use with caution if you have asthma.
- Taking n-acetyl cysteine with activated charcoal for poisoning may decrease its effectiveness.
- NAC increases the effect of nitroglycerin. Therefore, a person may develop a headache, dizziness, or lightheadedness with these two drugs are used together.
- NAC may slow blood clotting. Use with caution if taking a blood thinner or if you have a bleeding disorder.
- Since NAC may slow blood clotting, discontinue usage two weeks before surgery.

■ Conditions That Can Benefit from N-Acetylcysteine

- Acetaminophen overdose (given IV)

- Acute exposure to cyclopeptide containing mushrooms

- Acute liver failure

- Acute pennyroyal or clove oil ingestion-induced liver toxicity

- Alzheimer's disease

- Atelectasis

- Autism

- Before diagnostic bronchoscopy to aid with mucous plugging

- Bronchitis

- Carbon monoxide poisoning

- Carbon tetrachloride poisoning

- COPD (nebulized)

- Cystic fibrosis (nebulized) It works through cysteine-mediated disruption of disulfide cross-bridges in the glycoprotein matrix in mucus.

- Decreasing cisplatin-induced nephrotoxicity and salvage therapy in cisplatin kidney damage

- Drug-induced hearing loss (cisplatin and others)

- Dry eyes

- Hair loss

- Helps prevent nitroglycerin tolerance

- High homocysteine level

- Influenza

- Neuropathic pain

- Nitrate intolerance (used IV)

- Parkinson's disease

- Pneumonia

- Postoperative pulmonary care

- Post-trauma chest conditions

- Prevention of contrast-induced kidney damage

- Prevention of memory loss

- Protective effect on noise-induced hearing loss

- Schizophrenia

- Seizure disorder

- Stroke

- Topical treatment of keratoconjunctivitis sicca

- Tracheostomy care

- Trichotillomania (hair-pulling)

- Use to lower lipoprotein(a)

- Used in disorders of glutathione depletion

- Used in the early stages of pesticide-induced toxicity

Early research shows that NAC may be effective for the following conditions:

- Bipolar disorder
- Cancer
- Depression
- H. pylori infection
- Hepatorenal syndrome
- Necrotizing enterocolitis
- Sepsis
- Sickle cell disease
- Sjogren's syndrome

POMEGRANATE

The pomegranate (*Punica granatum L.*) is an ancient, unique fruit that grows on a small, long-living tree cultivated throughout the Mediterranean region, the Himalayas, in Southeast Asia, and in California and Arizona. The fruit of the *Punica granatum* (pomegranate) contains hundreds of phytochemicals. Pomegranate extracts have been shown to exhibit antioxidant properties, thought to be due to the action of ellagic acid, the main polyphenol in pomegranate. The tree/fruit can be divided into several anatomical compartments: (1) seed, (2) juice, (3) peel, (4) leaf, (5) flower, (6) bark, and (7) roots, each of which has interesting pharmacologic activity. The synergistic action of the pomegranate constituents appears to be superior to that of any single component.

Functions of Pomegranate in Your Body

- Aids in blood sugar regulation
- Anti-atherosclerotic
- Antibacterial
- Anti-carcinogenic (It exerts antiproliferative, anti-invasive, and antimetastatic effects, induces apoptosis through modulation of Bcl-2 proteins, increases p21 and p27, and downregulates the cyclin-cdk network.)
- Antidiarrheal (anti-parasitic)
- Antifungal
- Anti-hypertensive (both systolic and diastolic)
- Anti-inflammatory (It inhibits the activation of inflammatory pathways including NFk-B as well as other pathways.)
- Antioxidant
- Enhances exercise performance and recovery
- Free radical scavenger
- Immune modulation
- Inhibits COX-2

- Inhibits MAO-A enzymes (which catalyze the metabolism of monoamines such as norepinephrine, dopamine, and serotonin)
- Weakly estrogenic
- Wound healing

■ Conditions That Benefit from Pomegranate

- Alzheimer's disease
- Arthritis
- Bacterial infections
- Cardiovascular disease (prevention and therapy)
- Crohn's disease
- Diabetes
- Enhances exercise program and helps prevent muscle damage
- Hyperlipidemia
- Malaria
- Male infertility
- Menopause symptoms
- Obesity
- Prevention of cancer (experimental models of lung, colon, prostate, and skin cancer)
- Prevention of memory loss
- Rheumatoid arthritis
- Ulcerative colitis
- Ultraviolet radiation-induced skin damage

■ Recommended Daily Dosage

- Most common dosage is: 2 to 4 ounces (60 to 120 mL) a day
- Dose is higher for hypertension: 43 to 330 mL of pomegranate juice a day

■ Side Effects and Contraindications

- Any medications that affect the cytochrome P450 2D6 (CYP2D6) substrates in the liver may have an interaction with pomegranate.
- Since pomegranate lowers blood pressure, the patient may need to decrease their dose of blood pressure medication.
- Do not use if allergic to pomegranates.
- Since pomegranate affects blood pressure, discontinue use for two weeks before a scheduled surgery.

PYCNOGENOL

Pycnogenol is the trademarked name for a mixture of forty different anti-oxidants from the bark of the maritime pine tree (*Pinus maritime*). It is an oligomeric proanthocyanidins (OPC), which is one of the most common poly-phenolic substances. This supplement provides a variety of health benefits. It also may improve the effectiveness of Adderall in treating attention deficit disorder (ADD).

■ Functions of Pycnogenol in Your Body

- Blocks leukotrienes
- Elevates the body's production of glutathione and vitamin E
- Helps regulate nitric oxide production
- Improves endurance
- Improves the circulation in the capillaries
- Improves the immune function
- Increases the lifespan of vitamin C in the body
- Is an antioxidant
- Protects against platelet stickiness
- Relieves inflammation
- Stimulates natural killer cells

■ Conditions That Can Benefit from Pycnogenol

- Allergies
- Asthma
- Attention-deficit disorder (ADD) when used in conjunction with Adderall
- Diabetes
- Dysmenorrhea (painful menstrual cycles)
- Endometriosis
- Erectile dysfunction
- Gingivitis
- Heart disease
- Hepatitis C virus-associated type 2 diabetes
- Hypercholesterolemia
- Hypertension
- Immune building
- Improves athletic performance
- Jet lag
- Lupus
- Melasma
- Menopause
- Osteoarthritis
- Premenstrual syndrome (PMS)
- Retinopathy
- Rotator cuff tendonitis
- Skin ulcers

- Sunburn
- Tinnitus (ringing in the ears)
- Varicose veins
- Venous insufficiency

■ Recommended Daily Dosage

25 to 250 milligrams a day.

■ Side Effects and Contraindications

- Side effects are rare but may include gastrointestinal discomfort, headache, nausea, and dizziness.

- Using Pycnogenol along with herbs and nutrients that can slow blood clotting can increase the risk of bleeding in some individuals. These herbs and nutrients include angelica, clove, garlic, nattokinase, ginger, ginkgo, Panax ginseng, vitamin E, and others.

- Since Pycnogenol can affect clotting time, stop using Pycnogenol at least 2 weeks before a scheduled surgery and restart two weeks after surgery.

- Take Pycnogenol with or after meals since it has an astringent taste.

- Use with caution if you have an autoimmune disease since Pycnogenol may cause the immune system to become more active.

RESVERATROL

Resveratrol is a polyphenol that is fat soluble. It has numerous biological functions in the body. Resveratrol administration has increased the lifespans of animals fed a high-calorie diet, but it is not known whether resveratrol will have the same effects in humans. Resveratrol is contained in alcoholic beverages. Japanese Knotweed is a perennial plant native to Japan, Korea, and China. Japanese Knotweed is a common commercial source of resveratrol found in nutritional supplements. When taken orally, resveratrol is well absorbed, but its bioavailability is relatively low since it is rapidly metabolized and eliminated.

■ Functions of Resveratrol in Your Body

- Anti-inflammatory
- Anti-microbial
- Antioxidant
- Antiviral
- Cancer prevention
- Decreases platelet stickiness
- Improves bone health
- Increases HDL

- Increases SIRT1
- Induces phase II detoxification enzymes
- Inhibits COX-2 enzyme induction
- Inhibits mitochondrial reactive oxygen species (ROS) formation
- Inhibits oxidation of LDL cholesterol
- Lowers blood sugar and regulates hyperinsulinemia
- Opens arteries by increasing nitric oxide
- Phytoestrogen
- Protects endothelial function
- Stops the proliferation of cells that narrow arteries

▪ Conditions That Can Benefit from Resveratrol

- Cancer prevention and treatment
  - Colon
  - Pancreatic
  - Prostate
  - Stomach
  - Thyroid
- Cognitive decline/Alzheimer's disease
- Coronary heart disease
  - Controls the production of inflammatory lipid mediators
- Inhibits of both platelet activation and aggregation (clumping of platelets)
- Promotion of vasodilation (widening of blood vessels) by increasing the production of nitric oxide
- Hypertension
- Immune building
- Insulin resistance/diabetes
- Weight loss

▪ Recommended Daily Dosage

- 20 to 1,000 milligrams daily.
- Because resveratrol oxidizes easily, store it in a cool, dry place.

▪ Side Effects and Contraindications

- Resveratrol may cause any of the following symptoms if used in high doses:
  - Abdominal pain
  - Diarrhea
  - Flatulence
  - Nausea
- Do not use resveratrol if you have had a hormonally related cancer until more is known about the estrogenic activity of resveratrol.

◼ Food Sources

- Bilberries
- Blueberries
- Cocoa
- Cranberries
- Grape juice
- Grape skins
- Mulberries
- Peanuts
- Red wine

ROSEMARY

Rosemary (*Rosmarinus officinalis*) is a woody evergreen shrub that is native to the Mediterranean region but is now grown around the world for its culinary uses. This herb is high in many nutrients, including vitamins A, C, B_6, thiamine, and folate; minerals such as magnesium, calcium, copper, iron, and manganese; antioxidant compounds such as diterpene, carnosol, and rosmarinic acid; and essential oils. These components combine to make rosemary a powerful medicinal.

◼ Functions of Rosemary in Your Body

- Has anti-cancer properties
- Has anti-ulcer activity
- Improves digestion
- Improves estrogen breakdown
- Improves mood
- Increases bile flow
- Inhibits the bone breakdown associated with osteoporosis
- Inhibits weight gain
- Is an anti-inflammatory
- Is an antioxidant
- Is an antispasmodic
- Is antibacterial
- Is antifungal
- Is antiviral
- Lowers blood sugar
- Lowers cholesterol
- Protects the liver
- Protects the neurons and brain from ischemic injury (diminished blood flow)
- Reduces oxidative stress

◼ Conditions That Can Benefit from Rosemary

- Acne
- Addiction
- Alopecia (hair loss)
- Anxiety disorder

- Asthma
- Cancer
- Cardiovascular disease
- Cataracts
- Constipation
- Dandruff
- Depression
- Epilepsy
- Herpes simplex infection

- Hypercholesterolemia (high cholesterol)
- Insomnia
- Insulin resistance/diabetes
- Irritable bowel syndrome (IBS)
- Macular degeneration
- Memory loss (prevention and treatment)
- Pain control

■ Recommended Dosage

Rosemary is available in several forms:

- Liquid extract (45 percent rosemarinic acid): 1 to 4 milliliters, three times a day.

- Topical preparations (6 to 10 percent essential oil): Apply to the skin once or twice daily.

- Standardized extract: (6 percent carnosic acid, 1.5 percent ursolic acid, 1 percent rosmarinic acid): 200 to 800 milligrams daily.

■ Side Effects and Contraindications

Do not use rosemary if you have epilepsy, since this herb can induce seizures. Also avoid if you are trying to get pregnant, since rosemary can decrease fertility.

Rosemary can interact with a number of medications, from Lasix to lithium. Rosemary can also affect the ability of the blood to clot. If you have a bleeding disorder or are taking a medication or supplement that may thin your blood, do not take this herb. If you are planning to have surgery, discontinue this herbal therapy two weeks before the procedure. Speak to your healthcare provider or pharmacist to learn if any drugs you're taking might make it unwise to use rosemary.

Rosemary may decrease the absorption of iron, so use iron supplements at least two hours after taking rosemary.

If you are allergic to other members of the mint family, you may experience discomfort if you consume or topically apply rosemary to the skin. Reactions are typically mild.

Rosemary can cause side effects, including the following:

- Itchy scalp
- Muscle spasms
- Skin irritation
- Vomiting

THYME

Because of its distinctive taste, thyme (*Thymus vulgaris*) has long been a culinary staple. In recent years, thyme has also gained a reputation for its medicinal properties. This herb is packed with vitamins and minerals, including vitamin C, vitamin A, riboflavin, iron, copper, manganese, and more. It also contains phenolic antioxidants like zeaxanthin, lutein, and thymonin. But the most important substance responsible for the biological activity of thyme is thymol. Thyme essential oil contains 20 percent to 54 percent thymol, as well as the oils carvacrol, borneol, and geraniol. Together, these components give thyme important medicinal properties.

Functions of Thyme in Your Body

- Has antibacterial properties
- Has anticancer properties
- Has astringent properties
- Is an analgesic
- Is an antifungal
- Is an anti-inflammatory
- Is an antioxidant
- Is an antiparasitic
- Is an antispasmodic
- Is an antitussive
- Is an antiviral
- Is an expectorant
- Promotes good digestion

Conditions That Can Benefit from Thyme

- Build-up of dental plaque
- Common cold, bronchitis, laryngitis, and tonsillitis
- Candida vaginitis (vaginal yeast infection)
- Cough/bronchitis
- Diarrhea
- Gastritis
- Indigestion
- Rheumatological disorders such as arthritis
- Skin infections

■ Recommended Dosage

Currently, there is not enough evidence in humans to establish an optimally effective dose of thyme supplements. Please follow the manufacturer's directions on the tea, liquid extract, oil, and ointment containers, and speak to your healthcare provider.

■ Side Effects and Contraindications

Do not use thyme if you are allergic to the mint family. Also avoid during pregnancy.

Thyme can affect the ability of the blood to clot. If you have a bleeding disorder or are taking a medication or supplement that may thin your blood, do not take this herb. If you are planning to have surgery, discontinue this herbal therapy two weeks before the procedure. Speak to your healthcare provider or pharmacist to learn if any drugs you're taking might make it unwise to use thyme.

Thyme oil is usually safe when applied to the skin. Since there have been some reports of skin irritation, you should always test the thyme preparation on a small area of skin before applying it to a larger area.

The ingestion of thyme can lead to possible side effects, including the following:

- Convulsions
- Headache
- Vomiting
- Dizziness
- Nausea

WHITE WILLOW BARK EXTRACT

Derived from the bark of the white willow tree (*Salix alba*), white willow bark extract has been used for thousands of years as a medicinal. Chiefly, it is valued for its analgesic, anti-inflammatory, and fever-reducing effects. It is worth noting that aspirin owes its effectiveness to substances (salicylates) found in willow tree bark.

■ Functions of White Willow Bark Extract in Your Body

- Is an anti-inflammatory
- Reduces fever
- Is an antioxidant
- Relieves pain
- Prevents platelets from sticking together and forming blood clots

■ Conditions That Can Benefit from White Willow Bark Extract

- Fever
- Headache
- Low back pain
- Menstrual cramps
- Musculoskeletal pain
- Osteoarthritis
- Rheumatoid arthritis

■ Recommended Dosage

120 to 240 milligrams daily in divided doses.

■ Side Effects and Contraindications

If you are allergic to salicylates, do not use white willow bark extract. Since higher doses of white willow have blood-thinning effects, do not take this herb if you have a bleeding disorder or are taking a medication or supplement that may thin your blood. If you are planning to have surgery, discontinue this herbal therapy two weeks before the procedure. Speak to your healthcare provider or pharmacist to learn if any drugs you're taking might make it unwise to use white willow bark.

The possible side effects of this supplement include:

- Dizziness
- Nausea
- Rash
- Stomachache

CONCLUSION

Maintaining a robust immune system can be a challenge in today's world. Part 3 of this book, *Max Your Immunity*, has centered around herbal and nutritional therapies for immune building and decreasing inflammation.

Some of the nutrients are important to take on a regular basis and some are therapies to take when you are near individuals that have been sick and you want to maximize your immune system so that hopefully you do not contract the illness that they have. Some of these therapies have also been shown to shorten the course of the disease process if you have contracted it. In addition, new studies have shown that the development of tolerance, control of inflammation, and response to normal mucosal flora are interrelated and linked to precise immune mechanisms.

As you have seen, nutrients act as antioxidants and as cofactors at the level of cytokine regulation. Chronic nutritional and micronutrient deficiencies compromise cytokine response and affect immune cell trafficking. The combination of chronic undernutrition and infection further weakens the immune response, which leads to an alteration in immune cell populations and an increase in inflammatory mediators. Therefore, consider the nutrients and herbal therapies in Part 3 of book as possible additions to your own personalized immune building program.

Conclusion

An optimal immune system is your key to optimal health in today's world!

In Part 1 of this book, Max Your Immunity, you have learned how your immune system works. The immune system is classified into two different types: innate immunity and adaptive immunity. The purpose of both systems is to protect your body from disease or illness. You also examined autoimmune diseases in which your own immune system attacks one or more tissues or organs, resulting in functional impairment, inflammation, and sometimes permanent tissue damage. In addition, your immune system can change over time and not function as optimally as it once did.

Part 2 of this manuscript discussed the ten keys to maximizing your immune system.

- **Alcohol: Moderation Is the Key to Good Health.** Alcohol abuse negatively influences multiple pathways of the immune response, leading to an increased risk of developing infections.

- **Exercise: Whether You Like It or Not.** Exercising the right amount is three to four times a week, doubling your pulse for twenty minutes which has many positive effects upon the body. One of the little-known benefits of exercise is that it boosts your immune system by reducing chronic low-grade infection, improving various immune markers, and also improving your response to vaccinations.

- **Gut: A Healthy Gut Equals a Healthy Immune System.** Your gastrointestinal tract is literally 70 percent of your immune system. Therefore, if your gut is not healthy you are not healthy. The 5 R program for gut restoration: remove, replace, repopulate, repair, and rebalance is discussed to aid you in having a gastrointestinal tract that has the perfect microbiome mix to optimize immune function.

- **Inflammation: Its Effect on the Immune System.** Inflammation is a signal-mediated response to cellular insult by infectious agents, smoking, toxins, physical stresses, and even elevated cholesterol. Consequently, healthy immune systems use inflammation to fix an unbalanced body. A small amount of inflammation heals, too much inflammation is linked to many major diseases including having a negative impact on your immune system.

- **Sleep: Get a Good Night's Sleep.** A good night's sleep is paramount for proper functioning of your immune system. Chronic sleep deprivation can be seen as an unspecific state of chronic stress, which negatively impacts immune functions and your health in general. The adverse effects of chronic sleep deprivation comprise an enhanced risk for various diseases as a consequence of a persistent low-grade systemic inflammation, as well as immunodeficiency characterized by an enhanced susceptibility to infections and a reduced immune response to vaccination.

- **Smoking: How It Affects the Immune System.** Nicotine, which is one of the main constituents of cigarette smoke, suppresses the immune system.

- **Stress: Manage Your Stress.** Stress is an all-encompassing concept that comprises both challenging circumstances that are stressful along with both the psychological and physical response to stress. One of the major systems in the body that responds to demanding circumstances is the immune system. In fact, numerous facets of the immune system are associated with stress. When you are first stressed, within minutes the body prepares for injury or infection during what is called a "flight or fight" response.

  Likewise, both acute and long-term stress, which lasts for months or even years, are also associated with elevated levels of inflammatory cytokines but it has different consequences. Initially the body produces an inflammatory response to help the body heal and help the body eliminate pathogens. However, long-term inflammation causes dysregulation of the immune system and increases your risk of developing many other diseases.

- **Sugar: Minimize Your Sugar Intake.** Increased sugar compromises your immune system.

- **Thyroid: Optimize Thyroid Function.** As you have just seen, the thyroid hormone regulates most everything that goes on in the body which also includes the immune system. Growing evidence compiled over recent decades has revealed a two-way crosstalk between thyroid hormones and the immune system. Ideal thyroid function is a must in order to have, and preserve, optimal immune function.

- **Water: Stay Hydrated.** There is no substitute for water. The human body is comprised of 60 percent water.

Part 3 of this book explored how vitamins and trace elements counteract potential damage caused by reactive oxygen species (ROS) to cellular tissues as well as how they modulate immune cell function. Adequate intake of vitamins B(6), folate, B(12), C, E, and of selenium, zinc, copper, and iron supports a Th1 cytokine-mediated immune response with sufficient production of proinflammatory cytokines. This helps maintain an effective immune response and avoids a shift to an anti-inflammatory Th2 cell-mediated immune response and an increased risk of extracellular infections. Likewise, supplementation with these micronutrients reverses the Th2 cell-mediated immune response to a Th1 cytokine-regulated response with enhanced innate immunity. In addition, vitamin D plays an important role in both cell-mediated and humoral antibody response and supports a Th2-mediated anti-inflammatory cytokine profile. Furthermore, vitamin D deficiency is correlated with a higher susceptibility to infections due to impaired localized innate immunity and defects in antigen-specific cellular immune response.

Overall, inadequate intake and level of these vitamins and minerals may lead to compromised immunity, which predisposes you to infections. Herbal therapies were also discussed at length in this section along with examining medications, surgery to the intestinal tract, exposure to toxins, chronic stress, and the aging process all of which cause nutritional depletions compromising the immune system. Furthermore, infections themselves aggravate micronutrient deficiencies by reducing nutrient intake, increasing nutritional losses.

In short, it's important to recognize that you have the ability to protect yourself and your loved ones from many common diseases. By simply increasing your bodies' own built-in immune system, we all have the power to protect ourselves. Hopefully this book has provided you with several pathways to maximizing your immune system, in order for you, and the people you love, to achieve and maintain optimal health.

Resources

In this book, I've tried to provide all the information you need to create a program that will help you achieve and maintain the maximum immunity. Although you can put together and follow this regimen on your own, it is often helpful to work with a personalized medicine specialist and/or compounding pharmacist who can customize your program to your special needs. This can be especially important if you are managing a health condition and are already taking various medications. As you have learned in this book, certain diagnostic tests can also be valuable in helping you be healthy and stay healthy, finding the cause of your symptoms, and aiding your healthcare professional in developing a personalized medicine treatment plan, as well as guiding your supplement choices. Finally, whether you design your own regimen or rely on the guidance of a medical specialist or pharmacist, you will benefit most if you use pharmaceutical grade supplements, which meet the highest regulatory requirements. The following lists will guide you to the resources that can help you realize your goal of maximum immunity and good health.

FINDING A COMPOUNDING PHARMACY

Compounding is the practice of creating personalized medications to fill the gaps left by mass-produced medicine. To meet the special needs of an individual, a compounding pharmacy can provide unique dosages, innovative delivery methods, and unusual flavorings, and can also eliminate allergens and unnecessary fillers. Professional Compounding Centers of America can help you find a PCCA Member pharmacy in your area.

Professional Compounding
Centers of America
9901 South Wilcrest Drive
Houston, TX 77099
1-800-331-2498
www.pccarx.com

FINDING A FELLOWSHIP-TRAINED ANTI-AGING SPECIALIST

American Academy of Anti-Aging
Physicians
1510 West Montana Street
Chicago, IL 60614
1-773-528-4333
www.worldhealth.net

DIAGNOSTIC LABORATORY CONTACT INFORMATION

Medical testing now makes it possible to measure your amino acids, fatty acids, organic acids, vitamin levels, hormone levels, gastrointestinal function, genome, and much more. This means that your regimen can be personalized to meet your specific needs. The following laboratories can perform tests to evaluate many important aspects of your health. Before ordering any medical test, be sure to consult with your healthcare practitioner.

Cyrex Laboratories
2602 South 24th Street
Phoenix, AZ 85034
Phone: (877) 772–9739 (US)
(844) 216–4763 (Canada)
Website: www.cyrexlabs.com/

Doctor's Data
3755 Illinois Avenue
St. Charles, IL 60174
Phone: (800) 323–2784
Website: www.doctorsdata.com

Genova Diagnostics
63 Zillicoa Street
Asheville, NC 28801
Phone: (800) 522–4762
(828) 253–0621
Website: www.gdx.net

Genomind
2200 Renaissance Blvd., Suite 100
King of Prussia, PA 19406

Great Plains Laboratory
11813 West 77th Street
Lenexa, KS 66214
Phone: (800) 288–3383
(913) 341–8949
Website: www.greatplainslaboratory.
com/

**Microbiome Labs Research
Center**
1332 Waukegan Rd.
Glenview, IL 60025
Phone: 904-940-2208
Website: www.biomeFx.com

Rocky Mountain Analytical
105–32 Royal Vista Drive NW
Calgary, Alberta T3R 0H9
Canada
Phone: (866) 370–5227
(403) 241–4500
Website: www.rmalab.com

SpectraCell Laboratories
10401 Town Park Drive
Houston, TX 77072
Phone: (800) 227–5227
(713) 621–3101
Website: www.spectracell.com

ZRT Laboratory
8605 SW Creekside Place
Beaverton, OR 97008
Phone: (866) 600–1636
(503) 466– 2445
Website: www.zrtlab.com

PHARMACEUTICAL GRADE COMPANIES

You can find many good supplement brands at health food stores. Always make sure you buy pharmaceutical grade nutrients. The following pharmaceutical grade companies offer many quality nutritional supplements. Contact them for full product lists as well as for directions on ordering their products.

Biotics Research Corporation
6801 Biotics Research Drive
Rosenberg, TX 77471
Phone: (800) 231–5777
(281) 344–0909
Website: www.bioticsresearch.com

Body Bio
45 Reese Road
Millville, NJ 08332
Phone: (888) 327–9554 (toll free)
(856) 825–8338 (outside the US)
Website: www.bodybio.com

Designs for Health, Inc.
980 South Street
Suffield, CT 06078
Phone: (800) 847–8302
(860) 623–6314
Website: www.designsforhealth.com

Douglas Laboratories
112 Technology Drive
Pittsburgh, PA 15275
Phone: (800) 245–4440
Website: www.douglaslabs.com

Life Extension
5990 North Federal Highway
Fort Lauderdale, FL 33308
Phone: (800) 678–8989
Website: www.lifeextension.com

Metagenics
25 Enterprise
Aliso Viejo, CA 92656
Phone: (800) 692-9400
(949) 366–0818
Website: www.metagenics.com

Microbiome Labs
1332 Waukegan Rd.
Glenview, IL 60025
Phone: 904-940-2208
Website: microbiomelabs.com

Ortho Molecular Products
1991 Duncan Place
Woodstock, IL 60098
Phone: (800) 332–2351
Website: www.
   orthomolecularproducts.com

Vital Nutrients
45 Kenneth Dooley Drive
Middletown, CT 06457
Phone: (888) 328–9992 (toll free)
(860) 638–3675
Website: www.vitalnutrients.net

Xymogen
6900 Kingspointe Parkway
Orlando, FL 32819
Phone: (800) 647–6100
Website: www.xymogen.com

References

The information and recommendations presented in this book are based on the many up-to-date scientific studies, academic papers, and books. If the references for all these sources were printed here, they would add considerable bulk to the book and make it more expensive, as well. For this reason, the publisher and I have decided to present a complete list of references, categorized by chapter and topic, on the publisher's website. This format has the added advantage of enabling us to make you aware of further important studies and papers as they become available. You can find the references under the listing of my book at www.squareonepublishers.com

About the Author

Pamela Wartian Smith, M.D., MPH, MS, spent her first twenty years of practice as an emergency room physician with the Detroit Medical Center and then 26-years as an Anti-Aging/Functional Medicine specialist. She is a diplomat of the Board of the American Academy of Anti-Aging Physicians and is an internationally known speaker and author on the subject of Personalized Medicine. She also holds a Master's in Public Health Degree along with a Master's Degree in Metabolic and Nutritional Medicine.

She has been featured on CNN, PBS, and many other television networks, has been interviewed in numerous consumer magazines, and has hosted two of her own radio shows. Dr. Smith was one of the featured physicians on the PBS series "The Embrace of Aging" as well as the on-line medical series "Awakening from Alzheimer's" and "Regain Your Brain."

Dr. Pamela Smith is the founder of The Fellowship in Anti-Aging, Regenerative, and Functional Medicine and is the past co-director of the Master's Program in Metabolic and Nutritional Medicine, Morsani College of Medicine, University of South Florida.

She is the author of ten best-selling books, including *What You Must Know About Thyroid Disorders; What You Must Know About Vitamins, Minerals, Herbs and So Much More; What You Must Know About Women's Hormones;* and *What You Must Know About Memory Loss.*

Index

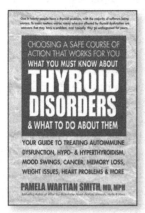

What You Must Know About Thyroid Disorders & What to Do About Them

Your Guide to Treating Autoimmune Dysfunction, Hypo- and Hyperthyroidism, Mood Swings, Cancer, Memory Loss, Weight Issues, Heart Problems & More

Pamela Wartian Smith, MD, MPH

It is estimated that one in twenty people have a thyroid problem, and that most sufferers go undiagnosed for years. But it doesn't have to be that way. Written by best-selling author Dr. Pamela Wartian Smith, *What You Must Know About Thyroid Disorders & What to Do About Them* enables readers to identify common thyroid problems and seek the treatment they need. The book begins by explaining the many functions that the thyroid performs in the body. It then goes on to discuss common thyroid-related disorders and symptoms, including hypothyroidism, hyperthyroidism, excess weight gain, thyroid cancer, and more. Finally, Dr. Smith explains each disorder's cause and common symptoms, diagnostic tests, and both conventional and alternative treatment approaches.

$16.95 US • 224 pages • 6 x 9-inch paperback • ISBN 978-0-7570-0424-7

What You Must Know About Women's Hormones

Your Guide to Natural Hormone Treatments for PMS, Menopause, Osteoporosis, PCOS, and More

Pamela Wartian Smith, MD, MPH

Hormonal imbalances can occur at any age and for a variety of reasons. While most hormone-related problems are associated with menopause, fluctuating hormone levels can cause a variety of other conditions. *What You Must Know About Women's Hormones* is a clear guide to the treatment of hormonal irregularities without the risks associated with standard hormone replacement

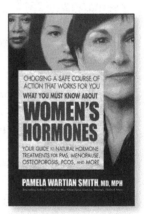

therapy. Part I describes the body's own hormones, looking at their functions and the problems that can occur if they are not at optimal levels. Part II focuses on common problems that arise from hormonal imbalances such as PMS. Finally, Part III details hormone replacement therapy, focusing on the difference between natural and synthetic treatments.

$17.95 US • 256 pages • 6 x 9-inch paperback • ISBN 978-0-7570-0307-3

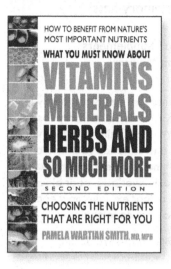

HOW TO BENEFIT FROM NATURE'S MOST IMPORTANT NUTRIENTS

WHAT YOU MUST KNOW ABOUT

VITAMINS MINERALS HERBS AND SO MUCH MORE

SECOND EDITION

CHOOSING THE NUTRIENTS THAT ARE RIGHT FOR YOU

PAMELA WARTIAN SMITH, MD, MPH

What You Must Know About Vitamins, Minerals, Herbs and So Much More
SECOND EDITION
Choosing the Nutrients That Are Right for You

Pamela Wartian Smith, MD, MPH

Almost 75 percent of your health and life expectancy is based on lifestyle, environment, and nutrition. Yet even if you follow a healthful diet, you are probably not getting all the nutrients you need to prevent disease. Why? There are many reasons, ranging from the mineral-depleted soils in which our foods are grown, to medications that rob the body of various vitamins and minerals. What, then, is the answer?

Now available in a fully revised edition that reflects the latest research and science-based studies, *What You Must Know About Vitamins, Minerals, Herbs and So Much More—Second Edition* explains how you can restore and maintain health through the wise use of nutrients. Part One of this easy-to-use guide presents the individual nutrients necessary for wellness. Part Two offers personalized nutritional programs for people with a wide variety of health concerns. People without prior medical problems can look to Part Three for their supplementation plans.

Whether you are trying to overcome a medical condition or you simply want to preserve good health, this new Second Edition can guide you in making the best dietary and supplement choices for you and your family.

ABOUT THE AUTHOR

Pamela Wartian Smith, MD, MPH, MS, is a diplomate of the American Academy of Anti-Aging Physicians and co-director of the Master's Program in Medical Sciences, with a concentration in Metabolic and Nutritional Medicine, at the Morsani College of Medicine, University of South Florida. An authority on the subjects of wellness and functional medicine, Dr. Smith is also the founder of the Fellowship in Anti-Aging, Regenerative, and Functional Medicine. Dr. Smith is also the best-selling author of seven books, including *What You Must Know About Women's Hormones; What You Must Know About Memory Loss;* and *What You Must Know About Allergy Relief.*

$16.95 US • 464 pages • 6 x 9-inch paperback • Health/Nutrition • ISBN 978-0-7570-0471-1

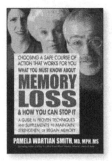

What You Must Know About Memory Loss & How You Can Stop It
A Guide to Proven Techniques and Supplements to Maintain, Strengthen, or Regain Memory
Pamela Wartian Smith, MD, MPH

Contrary to popular belief, not all memory loss is caused by the aging process. In *What You Must Know About Memory Loss & How You Can Stop It,* Dr. Pamela Wartian Smith describes what you can do to reverse the problem and enhance your mental abilities for years to come. You'll learn about the most common causes of memory loss, including nutritional deficiencies, hormonal imbalances, toxic overload, poor blood circulation, and lack of physical and mental exercise. The author explains how each cause is involved in impaired memory and supplies a list of proven remedies.

$15.95 US • 240 pages • 6 x 9-inch paperback • ISBN 978-0-7570-0386-8

What You Must Know About Allergy Relief
How to Overcome the Allergies You Have & Find the Hidden Allergies That Make You Sick
Earl Mindell, RPh, and Pamela Wartian Smith, MD

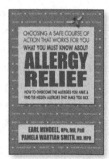

When most people have allergies, they know it. But for many others, allergies and intolerances are hidden culprits that lie at the heart of a number of health conditions. If you are an allergy sufferer or have a recurring health issue that you can't seem to resolve, this is the book for you. Written by a pharmacist and medical doctor, it provides important answers to common questions about allergies—what causes them, how they can affect you, and how you can overcome them. Up-to-date and easy to understand, *What You Must Know About Allergy Relief* offers the tools to identify hidden allergies and the means to relieve their symptoms.

$17.95 US • 288 pages • 6 x 9-inch paperback • ISBN 978-0-7570-0437-7

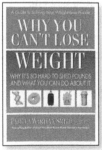

Why You Can't Lose Weight
Why It's So Hard to Shed Pounds and What You Can Do About It
Pamela Wartian Smith, MD, MPH

If you have tried to slim down without success, it may not be your fault. In this revolutionary book, Dr. Pamela Smith discusses the eighteen most common reasons why you can't lose weight, and guides you in overcoming the obstacles that stand between you and a trimmer body. It's time to learn what's really keeping you from reaching your goal. With *Why You Can't Lose Weight,* you'll discover how to shed pounds and enjoy radiant health.

$16.95 US • 256 pages • 6 x 9-inch paperback • ISBN 978-0-7570-0312-7